T0256908

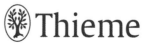

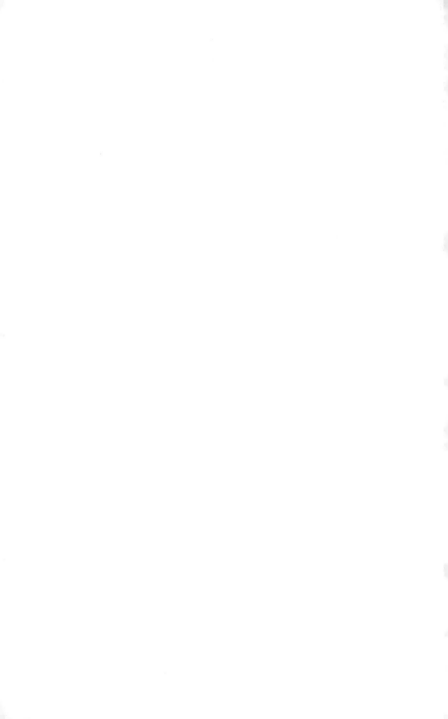

Pocket Atlas of Acupuncture and Trigger Points

Hans-Ulrich Hecker, MD
Private Practice
Kiel, Germany

Angelika Steveling, MD
Private Practice
Essen, Germany

Elmar T. Peuker, MD
Private Practice
Münster, Germany

Kay Liebchen, MD
Private Practice
Borgwedel, Germany

With contributions by

Michael Hammes, Stefan Kopp, Gustav Peters,
Beate Strittmatter

361 illustrations

Thieme
Stuttgart • New York • Delhi • Rio de Janeiro

Library of Congress Cataloging-in-Publication Data is available from the publisher.

This book is an authorized translation of the German edition published and copyrighted 2015 by Karl F. Haug Verlag, Stuttgart. Title of the German edition: Taschenatlas Akupunktur und Triggerpunkte

Translators: Ursula Vielkind, PhD, Dundas, Ontario, Canada; Johanna Cummings-Pertl, Hopland, CA, USA

Illustrator: Rüdiger Bremert, Munich, Germany; Helmut Holtermann, Dannenberg, Germany; Martin Wunderlich, Kiel, Germany

© 2018 Georg Thieme Verlag KG

Thieme Publishers Stuttgart
Rüdigerstrasse 14, 70469 Stuttgart, Germany
+49 [0]711 8931 421, customerservice@thieme.de

Thieme Publishers New York
333 Seventh Avenue, New York, NY 10001, USA
+1-800-782-3488, customerservice@thieme.com

Thieme Publishers Delhi
A-12, Second Floor, Sector-2, Noida-201301
Uttar Pradesh, India
+91 120 45 566 00, customerservice@thieme.in

Thieme Publishers Rio, Thieme Publicações Ltda.
Edifício Rodolpho de Paoli, 25º andar
Av. Nilo Peçanha, 50 – Sala 2508
Rio de Janeiro 20020-906 Brasil
+55 21 3172 2297 / +55 21 3172 1896

Cover design: Thieme Publishing Group

Typesetting by DiTech Process Solutions Pvt. Ltd., India

Printed in India by Replika Press Pvt. Ltd.

5 4 3 2 1

ISBN 978-3-13-241603-1

Also available as an e-book:
eISBN 978-3-13-241602-4

Important note: Medicine is an ever-changing science undergoing continual development. Research and clinical experience are continually expanding our knowledge, in particular our knowledge of proper treatment and drug therapy. Insofar as this book mentions any dosage or application, readers may rest assured that the authors, editors, and publishers have made every effort to ensure that such references are in accordance with **the state of knowledge at the time of production of the book.**

Nevertheless, this does not involve, imply, or express any guarantee or responsibility on the part of the publishers in respect to any dosage instructions and forms of applications stated in the book. **Every user is requested to examine carefully** the manufacturers' leaflets accompanying each drug and to check, if necessary in consultation with a physician or specialist, whether the dosage schedules mentioned therein or the contraindications stated by the manufacturers differ from the statements made in the present book. Such examination is particularly important with drugs that are either rarely used or have been newly released on the market. Every dosage schedule or every form of application used is entirely at the user's own risk and responsibility. The authors and publishers request every user to report to the publishers any discrepancies or inaccuracies noticed. If errors in this work are found after publication, errata will be posted at www.thieme.com on the product description page.

Some of the product names, patents, and registered designs referred to in this book are in fact registered trademarks or proprietary names even though specific reference to this fact is not always made in the text. Therefore, the appearance of a name without designation as proprietary is not to be construed as a representation by the publisher that it is in the public domain.

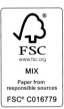

FSC
www.fsc.org
MIX
Paper from
responsible sources
FSC® C016779

Contents

Part 1
Body Acupuncture Points

Part 2

Ear Acupuncture Points

Part 3
Trigger Points

Part 4
Appendix

75   References   393

76   Illustration Credits   402

      Body Points   403
      Ear Points   407
      Trigger Points   411
      General Index   414

Preface

Acupuncture has developed into a recognized therapy option for many different disorders. Many universities have teaching positions for acupuncture. Even a few professorships for acupuncture and/or Chinese medicine have been established.

Acupuncture that meets the "lege artis" standard requires precise localization of acupuncture points. The concept we introduce for localizing acupuncture points based on given anatomical structures has established itself as a standard.

This pocket atlas contains three parts:

Part 1, Body Acupuncture Points, contains the most important points for body acupuncture and describes their location, depth of needling, indications and actions in Chinese medicine. A brief introduction presents the most important aspects of the history of body acupuncture and an overview of its mode of action.

Part 2, Ear Acupuncture Points, describes ear acupuncture points according to the Western school of acupuncture of Nogier and Bahr as well as according to Chinese teachings and explains the differences between them. This part also includes the latest findings and research on auricular innervation by Peuker et al.

Part 3, Trigger Points, introduces the most important defined trigger points of relevance in clinical practice, describes their relationship to corresponding acupuncture points, and discusses theoretical foundations.

We would like to thank everyone involved in the creation of this book, especially Ruediger Bremert and Helmut Holtermann for their excellent anatomical drawings. We are grateful to the entire staff at Thieme Publishers for their support in realizing this English edition.

Dr. Hans-Ulrich Hecker
Dr. Angelika Steveling
Dr. Elmar T. Peuker
Dr. Kay Liebchen

The Authors

Hecker, Hans-Ulrich, MD
Medical specialist in general medicine, naturopathy, homeopathy, acupuncture. Lecturer in Naturopathy and Acupuncture, Christian Albrecht University, Kiel, Germany.
Research Director of Education in Naturopathy and Acupuncture, Academy of Continuing Medical Education of the Regional Medical Association of Schleswig-Holstein. Certified Medical Quality Manager. Assessor of the European Foundation of Quality Management (EFQM).

Steveling, Angelika, MD
Department of Traditional Medicine and Pain Management, Grönemeyer Institute of Microtherapy, Bochum, Germany, Chair of Radiology and Microtherapy, University of Witten-Herdecke, Germany. Chiropractor, NLP practitioner, dietetic treatment.
Lecturer for continuing acupuncture education of the Regional Medical Association of Schleswig-Holstein.
Lecturer of the German Medical Association of Acupuncture (DÄGfA).

Peuker, Elmar T., MD
Medical specialist in internal and general medicine, medical specialist in anatomy, acupuncture, chiropractic, naturopathy, special pain management, and osteopathy. Certified health economist. Research Director of Education in Acupuncture, Academy of Continuing Medical Education of the Regional Medical Association of Westfalen-Lippe. Author and co-author of many books and articles.

Liebchen, Kay, MD
Medical specialist in orthopedics/rheumatology, chiropractic, physiotherapy, special pain management, sports medicine.
Instructor at the German Society for Chiropractic (MWE) and at the Academy for Osteopathy, Damp, Germany.
Lecturer for Acupuncture, Academy of Continuing Medical Education of the Regional Medical Association of Schleswig-Holstein, Germany, with a focus on combining acupuncture with manual therapy, osteopathy, trigger point therapy, and acu-taping. Author and co-author of many books and articles.
Chairman of the German Society for Acu-Taping.

Contributors

Hammes, Michael G., MD
Assistant physician, Neurological Clinic, Clinical Center Lippe-Lemgo, Germany. Acupuncture, special pain management. Post-graduate studies of TCM in China. Lecturer and board member of the German Medical Association of Acupuncture (DÄGfA).

Prof. Kopp, Stefan, DMD
Chief Physician and Director of the "Carolinum" Dental Institute, Orthodontic Outpatient Clinic, Clinical Center of the Johann Wolfgang Goethe-University, Frankfurt, Germany.

Peters, Gustav, MD
Medical specialist in general medicine, acupuncture, homeopathy, and chiropractic, Hankensbüttel, Germany.
Lecturer of the German Medical Association of Acupuncture (DÄGfA).
Focus on ear acupuncture/auriculomedicine.

Strittmatter, Beate, MD
Medical specialist in general medicine and sports medicine; naturopath and acupuncturist; Director of Education at the German Academy for Acupuncture and Auriculomedicine (DAA).

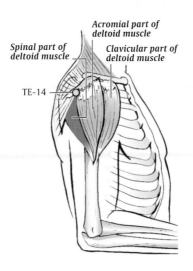

Spinal part of deltoid muscle

Acromial part of deltoid muscle

Clavicular part of deltoid muscle

TE-14

Part 1
Body Acupuncture
Points

1 Introduction

Body acupuncture originated in China and was first recorded in the literature about 90 BC. Initially, these records described five needle-insertion points on the lower arms and lower legs, which bore names analogous to the course of a running river:

- Well
- Spring
- Stream
- Channel (river)
- Uniting point

Even earlier, there existed wooden figurines with acupuncture channels, for example, those found in a grave from the Han Dynasty (200 BC to AD 9). According to traditional Chinese thinking, life energy, or Qi, circulates in these acupuncture channels, also called meridians.

Over time, more acupuncture points have been added to these channels and beyond. These are called extraordinary points. Current teaching includes 361 classic body acupuncture points.

The description and passing down of these acupuncture points probably follows empirical knowledge. For example, local points in especially painful areas were added and—if successful—retained and integrated into the system. This explains, for example, the more than coincidental correlation between acupuncture and trigger points. Other functions and combinations of points were added later based on observation or theoretical analysis.

Mechanisms of action on a segmental, or higher, functional level for treatment of pain disorders with acupuncture have been scientifically proven. Segmentally, acupuncture activates inhibitory interneurons via Aß fibers (A beta fibers, mechanoreception) and Aδ fibers (A delta fibers, rapidly conducting pain fibers). At a higher functional level, acupuncture causes the hypothalamic systems to produce endorphins that activate serotonergic and noradrenergic pathways.

There is also proof that acupuncture can inhibit the sympathetic nervous system and can activate the immune system. The connecting element here is most likely the hypothalamus–pituitary–adrenal system.

In the past, several attempts were made to define the anatomical correlations of acupuncture points. Initial work in this field came from the school of the Viennese anatomist G. Kellner, which postulated that acupuncture points are based on concentrations of certain receptors. However, it was not possible to provide specific proof of such concentrations.

In the 1980s, older research about acupuncture points was revisited, namely that they correspond to perforations in superficial body fascia by specific bundles of blood vessels and nerves. This theory is being tested primarily by a working group led by Professor Hartmut Heine. Other teams of researchers have also found that such fascia perforations are often located near acupuncture points. However, this does not provide specific proof, because such perforations are to be found in thousands of locations on the entire body.

Newer research (e.g., Dung, Peuker et al, Ma et al) indicates that the morphological correlation responsible for causing acupuncture effects may go beyond the structure reached by the tip of the needle. Given the varying effects of acupuncture, one can assume that the morphological substrates are also highly variable. This thesis is largely accepted in the English-speaking world, while the theory of fascia perforations is more common in the German-speaking areas.

The main target structures reached by acupuncture needles are—among others—septa, layers of connective tissue, and fasciae, as well as joint capsules, periostea, and epineural sheaths. These result in varying target theories for the effects of acupuncture.

Newer research shows a direct effect of needling on connective tissue fibers (Langevin). Considering the link between collagen fibers and cells that produce connective tissue via integrins, and the ability to influence the production and composition of the extracellular matrix, it becomes possible to build a stable bridge to the system of basic regulation (Pischinger and Heine) and therefore, connect acupuncture and classic natural healing methods.

2 Lung Channel

▶ Fig. 2.1

Major Points

- LU-1: Front collecting point (Mu Point)
- LU-5: Sedation point
- LU-7: Connecting point (Luo Point). Opening point of the Conception Vessel Ren Mai
- LU-9: Source point (Yuan Point). Tonification point, master point of the blood vessels
- LU-11: Local point

Associated Points

- LU-1: Front collecting point (Mu Point) of the lung
- BL-13: Back transport point (Back Shu Point) of the lung

Coupling Relationships

▶ Fig. 2.2

Top-to-bottom coupling: Lung–spleen

Yin-Yang coupling: Lung–large intestine

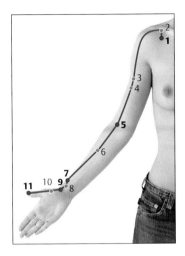

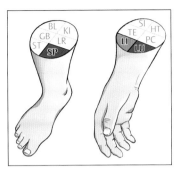

▶ **Fig. 2.2** Coupling relationships of the Lung Channel.

▶ **Fig. 2.1** Major points of the Lung Channel.

LU-1 Zhong Fu

"Central Treasury" ("Central Mansion"), Front Collecting Point (Mu Point)

Location: 6 Cun lateral to the median line, 1 Cun below the clavicle, slightly medial to the caudal border of the coracoid process, at the level of the first intercostal space (ICS 1) (▶ **Fig. 2.3**).

❗ Note

To locate the coracoid process, palpate in a cranial direction along the anterior fold of the armpit until you feel a distinct bony marker. The easiest way to palpate the coracoid process is by gliding the finger laterally at the caudal margin of the clavicle. Just before reaching the bony structure you are looking for, the finger slides into a soft depression (absence of bony ribs). The coracoid process is located laterally, slightly beyond that depression.

❗ Functional Note

Differentiation between the coracoid process and the lesser tubercle of the humerus: When the arm is rotated slightly outward with the elbow flexed, the coracoid process does not move, while the lesser tubercle of the humerus immediately follows the movement.

🔲 Practical Tip

LU-1 is located in the area of tendon insertions of the smaller pectoral muscle, biceps muscle of arm (short head), and coracobrachial muscle; these muscles are often shortened and sensitive to pressure in cases of poor posture in the thoracic region.

Depth of needling: 0.3 to 0.5 Cun.

This is one of the generally dangerous acupuncture points, because improper needling in the mediodorsal direction may create the risk of causing pneumothorax (e.g., in older patients with vesicular emphysema). To cause a pneumothorax, however, requires certain anatomical conditions and incorrect needling in the mediodorsal direction. This point should only be needled in the laterodorsal direction, that is, in the direction of the coracoid process, or tangential to the coracoid process.

Indication: Respiratory tract disorders, cough and bronchitis with phlegm, bronchial asthma, tonsillitis, shoulder–arm syndrome, thoracalgia (pain in the chest).

Action in TCM: Regulates the circulation of Lung Qi and in case of Lung Qi Stagnation.

LU-5 Chi Ze

"Cubit Marsh," Sedation Point

Location: Radial to the biceps tendon, in the elbow crease (▶ **Fig. 2.4**).

🔲 Note
Locating the biceps tendons is easiest when the lower arm is flexed and supine.

Depth of needling: 0.5 to 1 Cun, perpendicularly.

Indication: Bronchial asthma, bronchitis, croup, tonsillitis, epicondylopathia, skin disorders; possibly microphlebotomy in case of repletion disorders, possibly moxibustion in case of weakness (**caution**: asthma, ragweed allergy); pain and swelling on the inside of the knee; shoulder pain.

H. Schmidt: Repeated moxa in case of croup.

J. Bischko: For facial skin disorders.

Action in TCM: Expels Phlegm Heat from the Lung Channel.

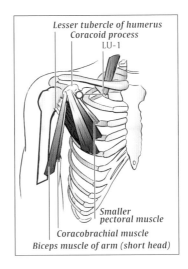

▶ **Fig. 2.3** LU-1.

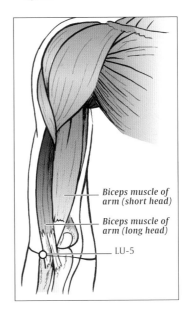

▶ **Fig. 2.4** LU-5.

LU-7 Lie Que

"Broken Sequence" ("Branching Crevice"), Connecting Point (Luo Point), Opening Point of the Conception Vessel

Location: Radiolateral on the lower arm, in a **V**-shaped groove proximal to the styloid process of the radius, 1.5 Cun proximal to the wrist crease (▶ **Fig. 2.5**).

! Note
This groove is created by the tendon of the brachioradial muscle, which inserts here at the radius, below the long abductor muscle of the thumb.

The tiger mouth grip may be used to find this point (▶ **Fig. 2.6**). LU-7 is located on the border between the inside and outside of the lower arm, right in front of the tip of the index finger.

As a point on a Yin channel, LU-7 still lies just within the Yin region.

! Note
To find this point: When using the tiger mouth grip, both practitioner and patient should keep the hand and lower arm of both arms straight and avoid bending or flexing the wrist.

Method of needling: Lift the skin to form a skin fold proximal to the styloid process of the radius, then insert the needle obliquely into the lifted fold in the proximal direction.

Depth of needling: 0.5 to 1 Cun.

Indication: Bronchial asthma, bronchitis, cough, wrist arthralgia, migraine, cephalgia, autonomic dysregulation, tics in the facial area, stuffy nose, facial paralysis.

Action in TCM:
- Regulates and descends Lung Qi
- Regulates Lung Disharmony caused by grief
- Clears the surface of pathogenic climate factors

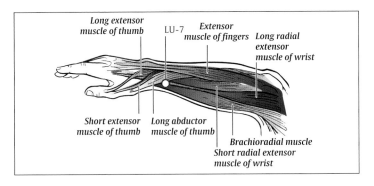

Long extensor muscle of thumb
LU-7
Extensor muscle of fingers
Long radial extensor muscle of wrist
Short extensor muscle of thumb
Long abductor muscle of thumb
Brachioradial muscle
Short radial extensor muscle of wrist

▶ **Fig. 2.5** LU-7.

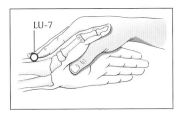

LU-7

▶ **Fig. 2.6** Tiger mouth grip.

LU-9 Tai Yuan

"Great Abyss" ("Great Gulf"), Source Point (Yuan Point), Tonification Point, Master Point of the Blood Vessels

Location: Radial side of the wrist flexion crease, lateral to the radial artery (▶ Fig. 2.7). Of the existing wrist creases, use the one running from the transition of the radius and ulna on one side and the wrist bones (carpal bones) on the other side. Select the wrist crease that is located distal to the clearly palpable end of the styloid process of the radius.

🅸 Note
The desired position of the needle is close to the radial artery. This results in a direct effect on the perivascular sympathetic neurovascular plexus. (Explanation of the effect of acupuncture according to König/Wancura: LU-9 is the master point for blood vessels.) The position of the needle is therefore correct when the needle pulses. From that point onward, however, there must be no more stimulation with the needle, that is, the sedation method must not be used. Accidental puncture of the radial artery has no effect whatsoever, as long as bypass circulation through the ulnar artery exists (to be established by prior palpation of the ulnar artery) and compression is subsequently applied.

Depth of needling: 2 to 3 mm, perpendicularly.

Indication: Respiratory tract disorders, bronchial asthma, chronic bronchitis, cough, circulatory disorders, peripheral arterial occlusive disease, Raynaud's disease, disorders of the wrist.

Action in TCM:
- Tonifies and replenishes Lung Qi and regulates its circulation
- Promotes circulation of Qi and Blood

LU-11 Shao Shang

"Lesser Shang" ("Young Shang")

Location: Radial corner of the thumbnail (Chinese), ulnar corner of the thumbnail (J. Bischko). As shown in the figure, the thumbnail corner point is located at the intersection of vertical and horizontal lines running along the bottom and side of the nail (▶ Fig. 2.8).

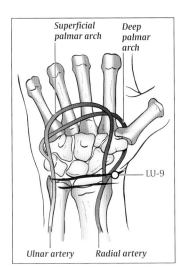

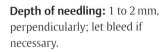

▶ **Fig. 2.7** LU-9.

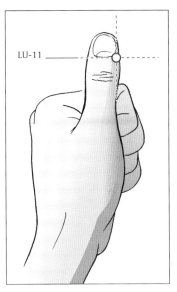

▶ **Fig. 2.8** LU-11.

Depth of needling: 1 to 2 mm, perpendicularly; let bleed if necessary.

Indication: Inflammatory throat disorders.

J. Bischko: Master point for throat disorders (see Additional Information (p. 23)), possibly with microphlebotomy in case of acute symptoms.

ℹ Additional Information

In addition to the eight proper master points (LR-13, CV-12 and 17, BL-11 and 17, GB-34 and 39, LU-9), J. Bischko described about 40 other "master points."

Action in TCM: Expels exterior Wind Heat.

3 Large Intestine Channel

▶ Fig. 3.1

Major Points

- LI-1: Local point
- LI-4: Source point (Yuan Point)
- LI-10: Local point
- LI-11: Tonification point
- LI-14: Local point
- LI-15: Local point
- LI-20: Local point

Associated Points

- ST-25: Front collecting point (Mu Point) of the large intestine
- BL-25: Back transport point (Back Shu Point) of the large intestine
- ST-37: Lower sea point (Lower He Point) of the large intestine

Coupling Relationships

▶ Fig. 3.2

Top-to-bottom coupling: Large intestine–stomach

Yang-Yin coupling: Large intestine–lung

LI-1 Shang Yang

"Metal Yang"

Location: Radial corner of the index finger nail (▶ **Fig. 3.3**); for exact localization of starting and end points of the channels of the hand, see LU-11 (p. 22).

Depth of needling: 1 to 2 mm, perpendicularly; let bleed if necessary.

Indication: Acute fever, acute toothache, acute inflammation of the throat; important analgesic point.

J. Bischko: Master point for toothache.

🛈 Additional Information

For more details on master points according to J. Bischko, see LU-11 (p. 22).

Action in TCM: Expels Heat and Wind Heat.

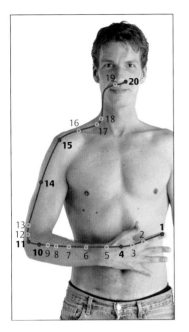

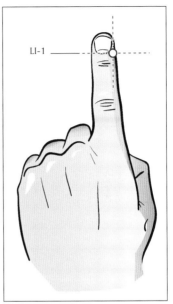

► **Fig. 3.3** LI-1.

► **Fig. 3.1** Major points of the Large Intestine Channel.

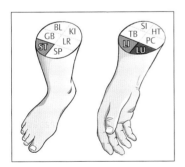

► **Fig. 3.2** Coupling relationships of the Large Intestine Channel.

LI-4 He Gu

"Union Valley" ("Connected Valleys," "Enclosed Valley"), Source Point (Yuan Point)

Location: There are several possibilities for localizing this most commonly used acupuncture point:

1. With thumb abducted, this point is located halfway on the line connecting the middle of the first metacarpal bone with the middle of the second metacarpal bone (▶ Fig. 3.4). The needle is pushed forward about 0.5 to 1 Cun toward the center of the lower surface of the shaft of the second metacarpal bone.

2. With thumb adducted, insert the needle into the highest point of the first dorsal interosseous muscle, which is contracted during adduction and pushed upward by the adductor muscle of the thumb (▶ Fig. 3.5). After inserting the needle, allow the hand to relax immediately and push the needle forward approximately 0.5 to 1 Cun toward the middle of the lower surface of the second metacarpal bone. This kind of localization can only be used when the highest point of the muscle bulge is located in the middle of the second metacarpal bone.

3. With thumb abducted, palpate in the direction of the second metacarpal bone with the flexed phalanx of the thumb of other hand. This localization aid serves particularly well for sensing the De Qi. The angled thumb is pressed moderately firmly against the lower surface of the second metacarpal bone. LI-4 in ▶ Fig. 3.6 corresponds to the deep localization of this point.

Depth of needling: 0.5 to 1 Cun, slightly oblique in a proximal direction toward the palm.

Indication: This is the most important analgesic point and affects the entire body; fever, beginning of feverish colds, hemiplegia, acne, eczema, disorders of the head region (pain, inflammation, allergic reactions), facial paralysis, abdominal symptoms, general stimulation of metabolism, stimulates labor, dysmenorrhea.

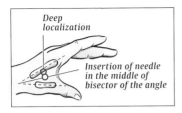

▶ **Fig. 3.4** LI-4 (1).

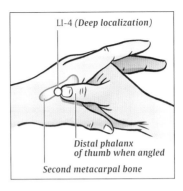

▶ **Fig. 3.6** LI-4 (3).

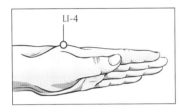

▶ **Fig. 3.5** LI-4 (2).

! Note

Do not perform downward (descending) stimulation during pregnancy.

Action in TCM:

- Expels exterior pathogenic climate factors
- Calms the Mind, consciousness (Shen)
- Regulates Lung Qi
- Removes Stagnation

LI-10 Shou San Li

"Arm Three Li" ("Hand Three Li")

Location: 2 Cun distal to LI-11 on the line connecting LI-5 and LI-11, in the long radial extensor muscle of the wrist (▶ **Fig. 3.7**); with deeper needling into the supinator muscle).

🔲 Note

Search for this point on a slightly flexed lower arm, with the thumb pointing upward.

Depth of Needling: 1 to 2 Cun, perpendicularly.

Indication: General tonification point (moxa); lateral humeral epicondylitis (tennis elbow), paresis of the upper extremity.
　H. Schmidt: Inflammatory facial rash, nasal furuncle (moxa).
　J. Bischko: Test point for obstipation.

Action in TCM: Removes obstructions from the channel.

LI-11 Qu Chi

"Pool at the Bend" ("Bent Pond"),
Tonification Point

Location: Lateral to the radial end of the elbow flexion crease when the lower arm is flexed at a right angle, in a depression between the end of the elbow crease and the lateral epicondyle, in the region of the long radial extensor muscle (▶ **Fig. 3.7**). This point is located between LU-5 and the lateral epicondyle of the humerus.

🔲 Note

If there are two creases, pulling the skin slightly toward the olecranon will identify the crease to be used.

Depth of needling: 1 to 2 Cun, perpendicularly.

Indication: Lateral humeral epicondylitis, paresis of the upper extremity, general immune-modulating effect, homeostatic effect, skin disorders, reducing fever; allergic disorders, abdominal disorders, soft or liquid stools with bad odor (traveler's diarrhea). Allow to bleed in cases of pharyngitis and laryngitis (hoarseness).

Action in TCM: Dispels Heat.

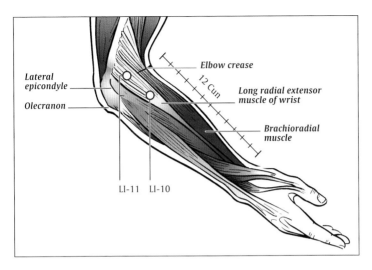

▶ **Fig. 3.7** LI-10 and LI-11.

LI-14 Bi Nao

"Upper Arm" ("Middle of Upper Arm")

Location: At the insertion of the medial part of the deltoid muscle. The point is located on the line connecting LI-11 and LI-15, 2 Cun caudal to the anterior end of the armpit fold (▶ **Fig. 3.8**). The insertion of the deltoid muscle can be easily localized when the arm is abducted.

Depth of needling: 0.5 to 1.5 Cun, perpendicularly.

Indication: Periarthritis of shoulder, neuralgia and paresis of the upper extremity.

Action in TCM: Removes obstructions from the channel.

LI-15 Jian Yu

"Shoulder Bone" ("Shoulder Blade")

Location: When the arm is abducted, two depressions are created slightly ventral and dorsal to the acromion. LI-15 is located in the area of the ventral depression, immediately below the ventral pole of the acromion (▶ **Fig. 3.8**).

ℹ Additional Information
The two depressions ventral and dorsal to the acromion have the following anatomical explanation:

The deltoid muscle consists of three parts:
1. The clavicular part.
2. The acromial part.
3. The spinal part (belonging to the spine of the scapula).

At each location on the shoulder girdle where two parts originate, a depression forms below the acromion, at the end of muscle grooves, which are often clearly visible.

❗ Note
The easiest way to find the ventral pole of the acromion is by laterally palpating along the ventral clavicular region. The dorsal pole of the acromion becomes palpable by following the scapular spine in a lateral direction.

Depth of needling: 0.5 Cun, perpendicularly, or 1 to 2 Cun oblique distal.

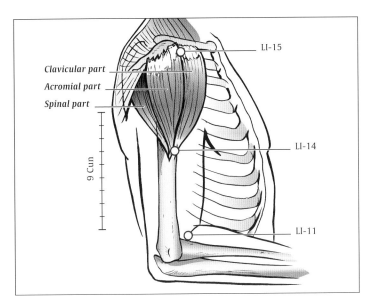

Clavicular part
Acromial part
Spinal part

9 Cun

LI-15

LI-14

LI-11

▶ **Fig. 3.8** LI-14 and LI-15.

🛈 Note
There is a risk of piercing the shoulder joint if needling in a vertical direction.

Indication: Periarthritis of the shoulder (frozen shoulder), paresis of the upper extremity, neuralgia of the upper extremity.

J. Bischko: Master point for paresis of the upper extremity (for more details on master points according to J. Bischko, see LU-11 (p. 22)).

H. Schmidt: In case of hemiplegia, daily moxa starting on day 7 after paralysis; prophylactic to prevent muscle atrophy.

Action in TCM: Removes obstructions from the channel.

LI-20 Ying Xiang

"Welcome Fragrance" ("Welcoming Perfume")

Location: Approximately 5 Fen lateral to the middle of the nasal wing, in the nasolabial groove (▶ Fig. 3.9).

Depth of needling: 3 to 8 mm, obliquely in a craniomedial direction.

> **🛈 Practical Tip**
> Cleanliness is particularly important in this region. Infected regions must *not* be needled under any circumstances. LI-20 is located close to the angular vein, which drains the blood from the facial area above the lips. The angular vein has an anastomosis to the ophthalmic vein and thereby is connected with the cavernous sinus. In the worst case, with infections, there is a risk of sinus thrombosis and central inflammatory processes.

Indication: Rhinitis, sinusitis, anosmia, toothache, facial paralysis, trigeminal neuralgia.

Action in TCM: Opens the nose, disperses Heat.

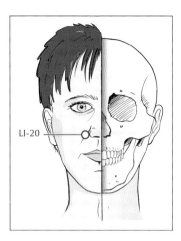

▶ **Fig. 3.9** LI-20.

4 Stomach Channel

▶ Fig. 4.1

Major Points

- ST-2: Local point
- ST-6: Local point
- ST-7: Local point
- ST-8: Local point
- ST-25: Front collecting point (Mu Point) of the large intestine
- ST-34: Cleft point (Xi Point)
- ST-35: Local point
- ST-36: Lower sea point (Lower He Point) of the stomach
- ST-38: Local point with remote effect on the shoulder
- ST-40: Connecting point (Luo Point)
- ST-41: Tonification point
- ST-44: Peripheral pain point

Associated Points

- CV-12: Front collecting point (Mu Point) of the stomach
- BL-21: Back transport point (Back Shu Point) of the stomach
- ST-36: Lower sea point (Lower He Point) of the stomach

Coupling Relationships

▶ Fig. 4.2

Top-to-bottom coupling: Large intestine–stomach

Yang-Yin coupling: Stomach–spleen

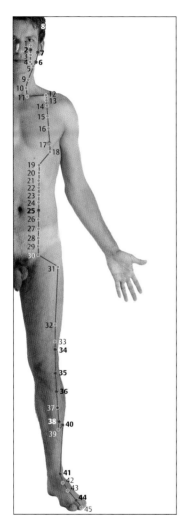

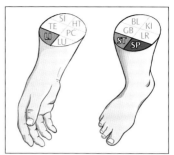

▶ **Fig. 4.2** Coupling relationships of the Stomach Channel.

▶ **Fig. 4.1** Major points of the Stomach Channel.

ST-2 Si Bai

"Four Whites"

Location: Above the infraorbital foramen, below the pupil when looking straight ahead (▶ **Fig. 4.3**).

🔲 Note
The infraorbital foramen is usually located slightly medial to the vertical line drawn through the middle of the pupil when looking straight ahead, approximately in the middle of the total length of the nose.

Depth of needling: 0.3 to 0.5 Cun, perpendicularly.

> 🔲 **Practical Tip**
> The risks resulting from needling in infected regions within the drainage area of the angular vein are as described for LI-20.

Indication: Eye disorders, migraine, rhinitis, sinusitis, facial paralysis, trigeminal neuralgia.

Action in TCM: Clears the eyes and supports vision.

ST-6 Jia Che

"Cheek Carriage" ("Mandibular Angle")

Location: 1 Cun cranial and ventral to the angle of the lower jaw. When biting down, a gap in the masseter muscle can be palpated in this location (▶ **Fig. 4.4**).

🔲 Note
The localization of ST-6 corresponds to that of a common trigger point in the insertion of the masseter muscle.

Depth of needling: 0.3 Cun, perpendicularly.

Indication: Myofacial pain dysfunction (temporomandibular disorder, Costen's syndrome), facial pain, facial paralysis, trigeminal neuralgia, toothache, gnathologic problems, teeth grinding.
   J. Bischko: Peroral skin efflorescence.

Action in TCM: Removes obstructions from the channel.

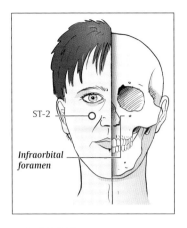

► **Fig. 4.3** ST-2.

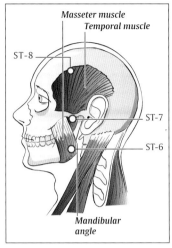

► **Fig. 4.4** ST-6.

ST-7 Xia Guan

"Below the Joint" ("Lower Pass")

Location: In the center of the depression below the zygomatic arch, in the mandibular notch between the coronoid process and the condylar process of the mandible. The condylar process of the mandible can be easily palpated in front of the tragus (it glides toward the front when the mouth is open). ST-7 is located in a depression immediately in front of it (▶ **Fig. 4.5**). This point is searched for and needled while the mouth is closed.

🔲 Note

Deep needling of this point reaches the lateral pterygoid muscle. Localization of ST-7 often corresponds to a trigger point in the lateral pterygoid muscle.

Depth of needling: 0.3 to 0.5 Cun, perpendicularly.

Indication: Myofacial pain dysfunction (Costen's syndrome), atypical facial pain, temporomandibular joint problems, facial paralysis, tinnitus, otalgia.

Action in TCM: Removes obstructions from the channel.

ST-8 Tou Wei

"Head Corner"

Location: 0.5 Cun into the hair from the frontal hairline, in the angle of this hairline with the temporal hairline running perpendicular to it (▶ **Fig. 4.6**).

Point ST-8 is located 4.5 Cun lateral to Point GV-24.

🔲 Note

Points ST-6, 7, and 8 lie approximately on a vertical line (▶ Fig. 4.4). If the original frontal hairline is no longer visible because of hair loss, it can be located by the patient frowning and identifying the border of the frontal folds.

Depth of needling: 2 to 4 mm, subcutaneously in a dorsal direction.

Indication: Cephalgia, migraine, eye disorders, atypical facial pain, vertigo.

Action in TCM: Clears Heat, eliminates Dampness and Phlegm in the head.

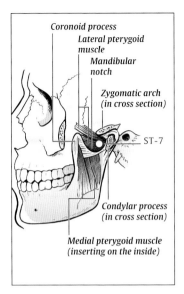

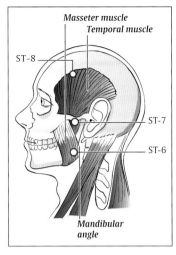

► **Fig. 4.6** ST-8.

► **Fig. 4.5** ST-7.

ST-25 Tian Shu

"Celestial Pivot" ("Upper Pivot"), Front Collecting Point (Mu Point)

Location: 2 Cun lateral to the navel (► **Fig. 4.7**).

Depth of needling: 0.5 to 1.5 Cun, perpendicularly.

Indication: Obstipation, meteorism, diarrhea, ulcers of the stomach and duodenum, Crohn's disease, ulcerative colitis, functional gastrointestinal problems.

Action in TCM: Eliminates Heat and Dampness in the intestine.

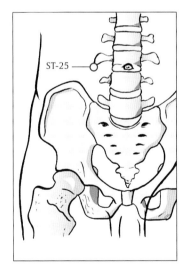

► **Fig. 4.7** ST-25.

ST-34 Liang Qiu

"Beam Hill" ("Hill Ridge"), Cleft Point (Xi Point)

Location: With the knee slightly flexed, 2 Cun above the lateral upper margin of the patella, in a depression within the lateral vastus muscle (▶ **Fig. 4.8**). This point is located on a line connecting the superior anterior iliac spine and the lateral upper pole of the patella.

❗ Note

All points of the knee region are searched for and needled with the knee slightly flexed (use padding to better support the patient).

Depth of needling: 1 to 2 Cun, perpendicularly.

Indication: Acute symptoms of the gastrointestinal tract, knee problems, nausea and vomiting; distant point used in mastitis.

Action in TCM:
- Descends rebellious Stomach Qi
- Clears channels, relieves pain

ST-35 Du Bi

"Calf's Nose"

Location: With the knee slightly flexed, below the patella and lateral to the patellar tendon

(▶ **Fig. 4.8**, ▶ **Fig. 4.9**); lateral "Eye of the Knee" ("Eye of the Knee" applies to the points caudal, medial, and lateral to the patella).

The lateral "Eye of the Knee" corresponds to Point ST-35, the medial "Eye of the Knee" corresponds to Extra Point Xi Yan (EX-LE-5).

❗ Note

Do not needle too deeply because of the risk of positioning the needle intra-articularly (within the joint). The lateral "Eye of the Knee" corresponds approximately to the location of arthroscopic access to the knee joint.

Depth of needling: 3 to 6 mm, in a slightly oblique medial direction.

Indication: Gonalgia.

Action in TCM:
- Removes obstructions from the channel
- Expels Wind and Cold

ST-36 Zu San Li

"Leg Three Li" ("Foot Three Li"), Lower Sea Point (Lower He Point) of the Stomach

Location: With the knee slightly flexed, 3 Cun below ST-35, approximately at the level of the

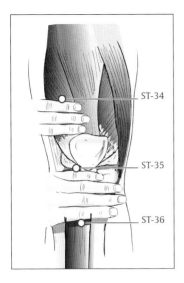

▶ **Fig. 4.8** ST-34 to ST-36.

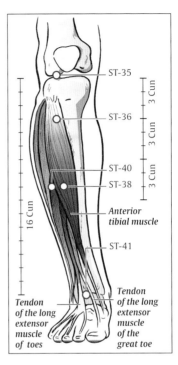

▶ **Fig. 4.9** ST-35 to ST-41.

lower border of the tibial tuberosity as well as about 1 Cun lateral to the tibial edge in the anterior tibial muscle (▶ **Fig. 4.8**, ▶ **Fig. 4.9**).

> **! Note**
> With dynamic palpating, a distinct depression is palpable at ST-36. In the German literature, the distance is usually given as 1 Cun lateral to the tibial edge, while Chinese literature always gives the slightly lesser width of 1 middle finger.

Depth of needling: 0.5 to 1.5 Cun, perpendicularly.

Indication: One of the most versatile and most frequently used acupuncture points (second to LI-4); a general tonification point, often used in moxa; homeostatic effect on metabolic disorders; distant point for abdominal disorders; strongly harmonizing effect on the psyche.

Action in TCM:
- Regulates Spleen and Stomach functional circles
- Tonifies/replenishes: whole body Qi and Defensive Qi (Wei Qi)

ST-38 Tiao Kou

"Ribbon Opening" ("Narrow Mouth")

Location: In the middle of the line connecting Points ST-35 and ST-41 (▶ **Fig. 4.10**), one width of the middle finger lateral to the tibial edge, or 2 Cun caudal to ST-37.

❗ Note
According to König/Wancura, the middle between the two points is best determined using the hand-span method. For this purpose, place the two little fingers on Points ST-35 and ST-41 and locate the center using both thumbs.

Depth of needling: 1 to 2 Cun, perpendicularly.

Indication: Distant point used in acute shoulder–arm syndrome.

Action in TCM: Expels Wind Dampness, relieves pain.

ST-40 Feng Long

"Bountiful Bulge" ("Rich and Prosperous"), Connecting Point (Luo Point)

Location: 1 width of the middle finger lateral to Point ST-38 (▶ **Fig. 4.10**).

Depth of needling: 1 to 2 Cun, obliquely in a medial direction.

Indication: Gastrointestinal disorders, hypersalivation (Dampness); "mucous disorders"—all disorders with excessive mucus production (mucous cough, mucous vomiting, mucous diarrhea).

Action in TCM: Drains Dampness, transforms Phlegm.

ST-41 Jie Xi

"Ravine Divide" ("Opened Hollow"), Tonification Point

Location: In the anterior middle of the line connecting the lateral malleolus with the medial malleolus, between the tendons of the long extensor muscle of the great toe and the long extensor muscle of toes over the upper ankle joint (▶ **Fig. 4.11**).

❗ Note
The tendon of the long extensor muscle of the great toe can be recognized by lifting the toe; Point ST-41 is located laterally. Deep needling reaches the upper ankle joint.

Depth of needling: 0.5 to 1 Cun, perpendicularly.

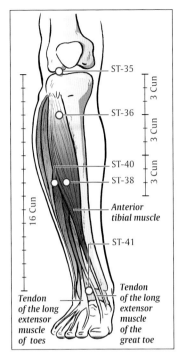

▶ **Fig. 4.10** ST-38 and ST-40.

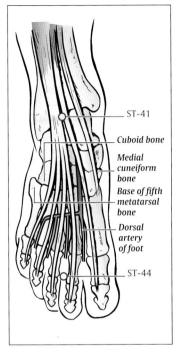

▶ **Fig. 4.11** ST-41 and ST-44.

Indication: Stomach problems, disorders of the ankle joint.

Action in TCM: Disperses Heat, calms the Mind (Shen).

ST-44 Nei Ting

"Inner Court"

Location: At the end of the inter-digital fold, between second and third toe (▶ **Fig. 4.11**).

Depth of needling: 0.3 to 1 Cun, perpendicularly.

Indication: An important pain point; frontal headache, nose-bleed, feverish colds.

    H. Schmidt: For upset stomach.

Action in TCM: Clears Heat, drains Heat.

5 Spleen Channel

▶ Fig. 5.1

Major Points

- SP-3: Source point (Yuan Point)
- SP-4: Connecting point (Luo Point). Opening point of the extraordinary channel Chong Mai (Penetrating Vessel)
- SP-6: Crossing point of the three Yin Channels of the foot
- SP-9: Local point with remote effect
- SP-10: Local point with remote effect

Associated Points

- LR-13: Front collecting point (Mu Point) of the spleen
- BL-20: Back transport point (Back Shu Point) of the spleen

Coupling Relationships

▶ Fig. 5.2

Top-to-bottom coupling: Lung–spleen

Yin-Yang coupling: Spleen–stomach

SP-3 Tai Bai

"Supreme White" ("Grand White," "Supreme Whiteness"), Source Point (Yuan Point)

Location: Inner side of the foot, proximal to the head of the first metatarsal bone, at the body–head transition of the first metatarsal bone (▶ Fig. 5.3), at the border between the side of the foot and the sole.

Depth of needling: 3 to 6 mm, perpendicularly.

Indication: General abdominal problems, lack of appetite, gastritis, vomiting, obstipation, diarrhea, meteorism, vertigo, chronic fatigue, sensation of fullness and tension in the thorax and epigastric region.

Action in TCM: Tonifies/replenishes the spleen.

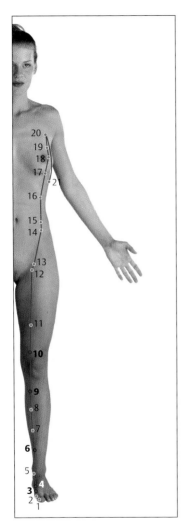

► **Fig. 5.1** Major points of the Spleen Channel.

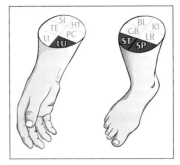

► **Fig. 5.2** Coupling relationships of the Spleen Channel.

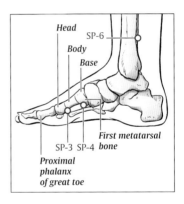

► **Fig. 5.3** SP-3.

SP-4 Gong Sun

"Yellow Emperor" ("Collateral Point of Spleen Channel," "Grandfather Grandson"), Connecting Point (Luo Point), Opening Point of the Extraordinary Channel Chong Mai (Penetrating Vessel)

Location: In a depression at the body–base transition of the first metatarsal bone (▶ Fig. 5.4), at the border between the side of the foot and the sole.

Depth of needling: 0.5 to 1 Cun, perpendicularly.

Indication: Stomach problems, Roemheld Syndrome (gastrocardiac syndrome), loss of appetite, indigestion with thin bowel movements, dysmenorrhea.
   J. Bischko: Master point for diarrhea.

Action in TCM:
- Tonifies/replenishes the spleen and stomach
- Regulates the Penetrating Vessel (Chong Mai) and menstruation

SP-6 San Yin Jiao

"Three Yin Intersection" ("Crossroad of Three Yins"), Crossing Point of the Three Yin Channels of the Foot

Location: 3 Cun above the largest prominence of the medial malleolus, at the posterior tibial edge (▶ Fig. 5.5), in a depression often clearly palpable (particularly in women).
   Occasionally, this point may be located slightly more to the front, in the tibial region.

Depth of needling: 1 to 2 Cun, perpendicularly.

Indication: The third most common acupuncture point; a general tonification point (moxa); "Royal Point" for all gynecological problems; facilitation of birth; acceleration of uterine contractions, gastrointestinal disorders, urogenital disorders (erectile dysfunction, female sexual dysfunction, dysmenorrhea); also effective in allergic and immunological disorders; skin disorders.
   König/Wancura: Basic point, in combination with Point HT-7, for treating psychosomatic disorders.
   Basic point, in combination with Point CV-4, for urogenital tract disorders.

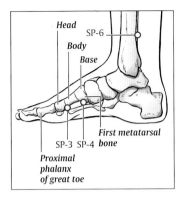

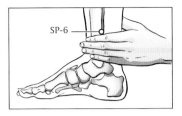

► **Fig. 5.5** SP-6.

► **Fig. 5.4** SP-4.

🛈 Note
Caution is recommended,
especially in early and late
pregnancy.

Action in TCM:

- Tonifies/replenishes:
  - Spleen
  - Blood and Yin
- Regulates
  - Menstruation
  - Qi and blood flow, relieves
    pain in the lower abdomen
- Sedates/calms the Mind (Shen)

SP-9 Yin Ling Quan

"Yin Mound Spring" ("Yin Hill Fountain")

Location: In the depression distal to the medial condyle of the tibia, at the transition from the medial condyle to the body of the tibia, in front of the belly of the gastrocnemius muscle (▶ **Fig. 5.6**) at the same level as Point GB-34.

Depth of needling: 0.5 to 1 Cun, perpendicularly.

Indication: Main point for eliminating accumulations of water and moisture, especially in the lower half of the body, micturition problems, dysuria, urinary tract infections, dysmenorrhea, vaginal discharge, fetid diarrhea, abdominal spasm, gonalgia, arthritis of the knee joints.

    H. Schmidt: Enuresis (moxa).

Action in TCM: Transforms Dampness.

SP-10 Xue Hai

"Sea of Blood" ("Blood Sea")

Location: With the knee flexed, 2 Cun proximal to the medial cranial pole of the patella, on the medial vastus muscle, in an often clearly palpable depression (▶ **Fig. 5.7**). Another way to locate this point is to place the palm onto the patella with the thumb slightly abducted; Point SP-10 is located in front of the tip of the thumb (▶ **Fig. 5.8**).

Depth of needling: 1 to 2 Cun, perpendicularly.

Indication: Important immuno-modulation point (together with Point LI-11).

    Skin disorders, pruritus, urogenital tract disorders, dysmenorrhea.

Action in TCM:
- Regulates Blood and removes Blood Stasis
- Cools Blood and stops bleeding

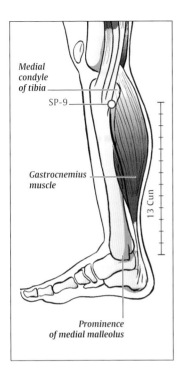

▶ **Fig. 5.6** SP-9.

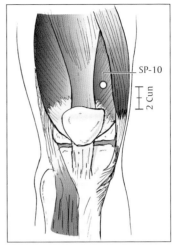

▶ **Fig. 5.7** SP-10 (1).

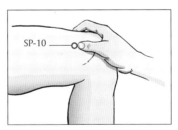

▶ **Fig. 5.8** SP10 (2).

6 Heart Channel

▶ Fig. 6.1

Major Points

- HT-3: Local point with general effect
- HT-5: Connecting point (Luo Point)
- HT-7: Source point (Yuan Point), sedation point

Associated Points

- CV-14: Front collecting point (Mu Point) of the heart
- BL-15: Back transport point (Back Shu Point) of the heart

Coupling Relationships

▶ Fig. 6.2

Top-to-bottom coupling: Heart–kidney

Yin-Yang coupling: Heart–small intestine

HT-3 Shao Hai

"Lesser Sea" ("Young Sea")

Location: With elbow flexed, between the ulnar end of the elbow flexion crease and the medial epicondyle of the humerus (▶ **Fig. 6.3**).

Depth of needling: 0.5 to 1 Cun, perpendicularly.

Indication: "Joy of Life," psycho-vegetative dysregulation, sleep disorders, mental agitation (Heart Fire, use sedative stimulation during the acute phase), depressive mood (caution when using the sedation method), vertigo, medial humeral epicondylitis (golfer's elbow), hand tremor.

Action in TCM: Calms the Mind (Shen).

HT-5 Tong Li

"Connecting Li," Connecting Point (Luo Point)

Location: 1 Cun proximal to HT-7, radial to the tendon of the ulnar flexor muscle of the wrist (▶ **Fig. 6.3**).

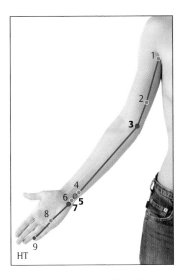

▶ **Fig. 6.1** Major points of the Heart Channel.

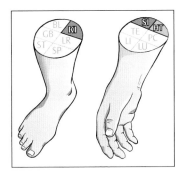

▶ **Fig. 6.2** Coupling relationships of the Heart Channel.

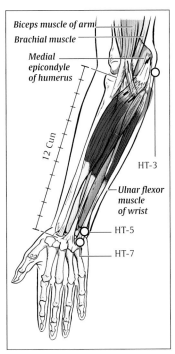

▶ **Fig. 6.3** HE-3 and HE-5.

Depth of needling: Up to 0.5 Cun, perpendicularly.

Indication: Psychovegetative dysregulation, functional heart problems, examination anxiety, anxiety attacks and restlessness, sleep disorders, sweating.

Action in TCM: Strengthens Heart Qi and Heart Yin.

HT-7 Shen Men

"Spirit Gate" ("Spiritual Gate"), Source Point (Yuan Point), Sedation Point

Location: At the flexion crease of the wrist, radial to the tendon of the ulnar flexor muscle of the wrist (▶ **Fig. 6.4**).

> **!** Note
> The flexion crease required for localizing this point lies between the radius and ulna on the one side and the wrist bones (carpal bones) on the other. The pisiform bone clearly marks this region in an ulnar direction. Therefore, use the flexion crease of the wrist lying proximal to the pisiform bone.

According to many descriptions in the German literature, a second possibility for needling this point is from the ulnar side. The direction of needling here is parallel to the flexion crease of the wrist; that is, at an angle of 90° relative to the needling method described above. The tip of the needle then lies dorsal to the tendon of the ulnar flexor muscle of the wrist. HT-7 is located deeply, where the tips of the two needles would meet if coming from volar and ulnar directions (▶ **Fig. 6.5**). This direction of needling, however, is not known in the Chinese literature.

Depth of needling: 0.3 to 0.5 Cun, perpendicularly, from a volar or ulnar direction.

Indication: Sleep disorders, anxiety attacks, circulatory dysregulation, withdrawal symptoms during addiction therapy, hyperactivity.

König/Wancura: Backbone for the treatment of psychosomatic disorders, in combination with Point SP-6.

Action in TCM:
- Harmonizes the Mind (Shen)
- Nourishes Heart Blood
- Regulates the Heart

> **!** Note
> Select your stimulation method carefully; sedate Point HT-7 only in case of confirmed repletion syndromes; watch for red tip of the tongue (e.g., Heart Heat).

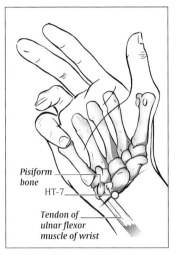

▶ **Fig. 6.4** HE-7 (1).

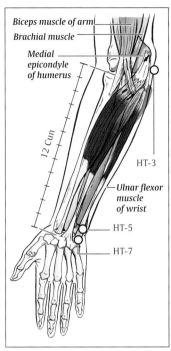

▶ **Fig. 6.5** HE-7 (2).

7 Small Intestine Channel

▶ Fig. 7.1, ▶ Fig. 7.2

Major Points

- SI-3: Tonification point. Opening point of the Governing Vessel, Du Mai
- SI-8: Sedation point
- SI-11: Local point
- SI-12: Local point
- SI-14: Local point
- SI-18: Local point
- SI-19: Local point

Associated Points

- CV-4: Front collecting point (Mu Point) of the small intestine

- BL-27: Back transport point (Back Shu Point) of the small intestine
- ST-39: Lower sea point (Lower He Point) of the small intestine

Coupling Relationships

▶ Fig. 7.3

Top-to-bottom coupling: Small intestine–bladder

Yang-Yin coupling: Small intestine–heart

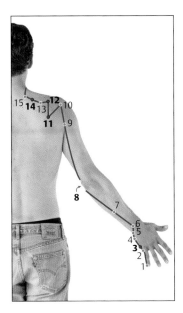

▶ **Fig. 7.1** Major points of the Small Intestine Channel (1)

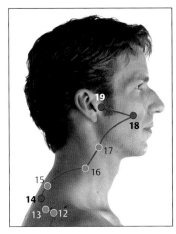

▶ **Fig. 7.2** Major points of the Small Intestine Channel (2).

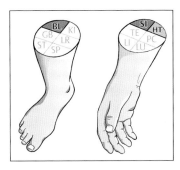

▶ **Fig. 7.3** Coupling Relationships of the Small Intestine Channel.

SI-3 Hou Xi

"Back Ravine," Tonification Point, Opening Point of the Governing Vessel, Du Mai

Location: At the ulnar edge of the hand, with a loosely closed fist, proximal and dorsal to a skin fold at the ulnar end of the most distal flexion crease of the palm. This point is located at the body–head transition of the fifth metacarpal bone (Gleditsch, König/Wancura) (▶ **Fig. 7.4**).

❗ Note
With a loosely closed fist, follow the distal flexion crease of the palm in the ulnar direction. It usually starts between index and middle fingers. At the end of the flexion crease is a small bulge of skin. Point SI-3 is located at the border of this bulge and the surrounding area, slightly proximal and dorsal. Direct the needle toward the middle of the palm.

According to Chinese literature, this point is localized at the distal end of the flexion crease described, at the border between the side of the hand and the palm. Needling takes place in a vertical direction. With the localization method described in the previous paragraph, needling takes place in a slightly distal direction. These two slightly different localizations of this point meet in the deep, where the De Qi sensation originates. In our experience, the localization given by Gleditsch, which is also described by König/Wancura, has proved more effective for diagnosis and therapy.

Depth of needling: 0.5 to 1 Cun in the direction of the palm.

Indication: Acute lumbago, lumbago–sciatica syndrome (sciatica or sciatic neuralgia); distant point for the cervical spine; torticollis, paresis of the upper extremity, tinnitus, hearing loss, ear disorders, feverish colds, pharyngitis, laryngitis, tremor, vertigo.
  J. Bischko: The main indication for this point is spasmolysis.

🛈 Practical Tip
With acute torticollis, acute lumbago, or lumbago–sciatica syndrome (sciatica or sciatic neuralgia), treatment is followed by vigorous stimulation of Point SI-3 only, along with careful physical exercise.

Action in TCM:
- Opens the channels and network vessels (Luo) and relieves pain
- Supports the neck, back of the head, and back

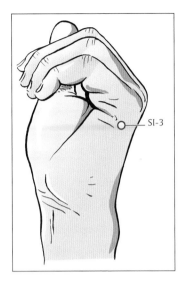

▶ **Fig. 7.4** SI-3.

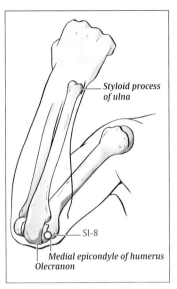

Styloid process of ulna

Medial epicondyle of humerus
Olecranon

SI-8

▶ **Fig. 7.5** SI-8.

SI-8 Xiao Hai

"Small Sea," Sedation Point

Location: When the arm is flexed, in the ulnar sulcus between the olecranon and medial epicondyle of the humerus (▶ **Fig. 7.5**).

Depth of needling: 4 to 8 mm, perpendicularly.

🚱 Practical Tip

SI-8 is located in close proximity to the ulnar nerve, which might be accidentally needled. If this happens, withdraw the needle immediately, but do not remove it completely.

Indication: Medial humeral epicondylitis (golfer's elbow); pain in the throat, shoulder, and neck regions.

Action in TCM: Removes obstructions from the channel.

SI-11 Tian Zong

"Celestial Gathering" ("Celestial Watching")

Location: In the infraspinous fossa, on a line connecting the middle of the clearly palpable scapular spine and the inferior angle of the scapula. SI-11 is located on this line at the transition from the cranial third and the remaining two-thirds. It is located immediately below SI-12, at the level of the lower edge of the spinous process of T4 and forms a triangle with SI-9 and SI-10 (▶ **Fig. 7.6**).

Depth of needling: 0.5 to 1 Cun, perpendicularly.

Indication: Pain and loss of motion in the shoulder (especially on exterior rotation), tightness in the thorax; in combination with other points for lactation disorders and mastitis.
 H. Schmidt: Special point for insufficient lactation.

Action in TCM: Removes obstructions from the channel.

SI-12 Bing Feng

"Grasping the Wind"

Location: Perpendicular to and above SI-11, approximately 1 Cun above the middle of the cranial border of the scapular spine (▶ **Fig. 7.6**). This point forms a triangle with Points SI-10 and SI-11. Common trigger point in the supraspinatus muscle.

Depth of needling: 0.5 to 1 Cun, perpendicularly.

Indication: Pain and loss of motion in the shoulder (especially on abduction and exterior rotation), supraspinatus syndrome, pain and paresthesia of the upper extremity, stiff neck.

Action in TCM: Removes obstructions from the channel.

SI-14 Jian Wai Shu

"Outer Shoulder Transport" ("Exterior Shoulder")

Location: 3 Cun lateral to the spinous process of T1 (▶ **Fig. 7.6**).
 Common trigger point in the levator muscle of the scapula.

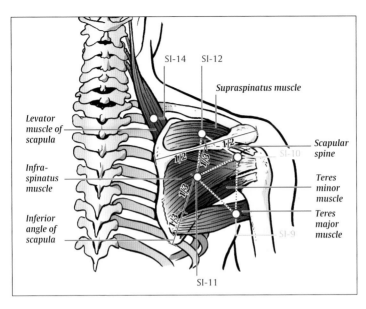

▶ **Fig. 7.6** SI-11, SI-12, and SI-14.

Depth of needling: 0.5 to 1 Cun, perpendicularly.

Indication: Pain and loss of motion in the shoulder, stiff neck.

🔲 Note

With the patient's arms hanging down, the distance of the dorsal median line through the spinous process and the medial border of the spine of the scapula is 3 Cun.

Action in TCM: Removes obstructions from the channel.

SI-18 Quan Liao

"Cheek Bone-Hole" ("Cheek Crevice")

Location: At the lower edge of the zygomatic arch, perpendicular to and below the outer corner of the eye, at the anterior margin of the masseter muscle (▶ Fig. 7.7).

🛈 Note

The anterior margin of the masseter muscle is clearly palpable during chewing.

Depth of needling: 0.3 to 0.5 Cun, perpendicularly.

Indication: Myofacial pain dysfunction (temporomandibular disorder, Costen's syndrome), trigeminal neuralgia, facial spasm, facial paresis, toothache, maxillary sinusitis, gnathologic problems.

Action in TCM:
- Expels Wind and relieves pain
- Clears Heat

SI-19 Ting Gong

"Auditory Palace"

Location: In the depression in front of the tragus (▶ Fig. 7.7, ▶ Fig. 7.8).

🛈 Note

Localize this point with the patient's mouth slightly opened. This causes the condylar process of the mandible of the temporomandibular joint to move in a nasal direction and prevents the risk of needling the temporomandibular joint. After inserting the needle, the mouth is closed again.

🗲 Practical Tip

SI-19 is located in the immediate proximity of the superficial temporal artery. This artery can be avoided by palpating the pulse prior to needling.

Depth of needling: 0.3 to 0.5 Cun, perpendicularly.

Indication: Ear disorders, facial paresis, trigeminal neuralgia, myofacial pain dysfunction (Costen's syndrome), temporomandibular joint dysfunction.

Action in TCM:
- Promotes hearing
- Eliminates Wind

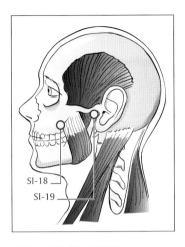

▶ **Fig. 7.7** SI-18 and SI-19.

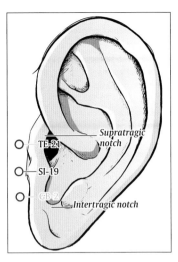

▶ **Fig. 7.8** SI-19.

8 Bladder Channel

▶ Fig. 8.1, ▶ Fig. 8.2

Major Points

- BL-2: Local point
- BL-10: Influences the parasympathetic nervous system
- BL-11: Master point of the bones
- BL-13: Back Shu Point of the lung
- BL-14: Back Shu Point of the pericardium
- BL-15: Back Shu Point of the heart
- BL-17: Back Shu Point of the diaphragm. "Master Point of the blood"
- BL-18: Back Shu Point of the liver
- BL-19: Back Shu Point of the gallbladder
- BL-20: Back Shu Point of the spleen
- BL-21: Back Shu Point of the stomach
- BL-23: Back Shu Point of the kidney
- BL-25: Back Shu Point of the large intestine
- BL-27: Back Shu Point of the small intestine
- BL-28: Back Shu Point of the bladder
- BL-36: Local point with a wide spectrum of activity
- BL-40: Lower sea point (Lower He Point) of the bladder
- BL-43: Wide spectrum of activity
- BL-54: Local point
- BL-57: Local point
- BL-60: Peripheral pain point
- BL-62: Opening point of the extraordinary channel, Yang Qiao Mai (Yang Heel Vessel)
- BL-67: Tonification point

Associated Points

- CV-3: Front collecting point (Mu Point) of the bladder
- BL-28: Back transport point (Back Shu Point) of the bladder
- BL-40: Lower sea point (Lower He Point) of the bladder

Coupling Relationships

▶ Fig. 8.3

Top-to-bottom coupling: Small intestine–bladder

Yang-Yin coupling: Bladder–kidney

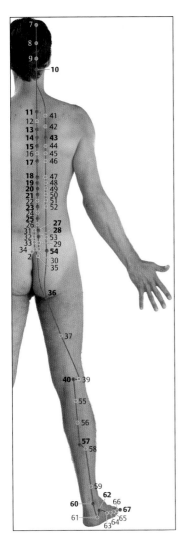

▶ **Fig. 8.1** Major points of the Bladder Channel (1).

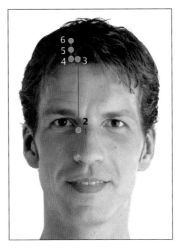

▶ **Fig. 8.2** Major points of the Bladder Channel (2).

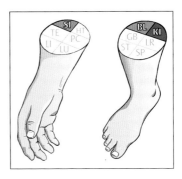

▶ **Fig. 8.3** Coupling relationships of the Bladder Channel.

BL-2 Zan Zhu

"Bamboo Gathering" ("Gathering Eyebrows")

Location: At the medial end of the eyebrow, above the inner corner of the eye. This point is located over the medial frontal notch at the edge of the orbit, which is often palpable (▶ **Fig. 8.4**).

Depth of needling: Approximately 0.3 Cun, subcutaneously toward the root of the nose or caudally in the direction of BL-1.

ℹ️ Note

The frontal notch represents the exit of the supratrochlear artery and the medial branch of the supraorbital nerve. It is not the supraorbital foramen, which is clearly further laterally and represents the exit of both the supraorbital artery and the lateral branch of the supraorbital nerve. Both points of exit can vary in shape and position. The frontal notch rarely appears as the frontal foramen; the supraorbital foramen rarely appears as the supraorbital notch.

ℹ️ Additional Information

Chinese literature mentions a "supraorbital notch" through which the medial branch of the supraorbital nerve passes. This notch is not the same as the supraorbital foramen.

Indication: Eye disorders, cephalgia, nasal pharynx disorders, pollinosis, urge to sneeze, glaucoma, dry eye syndrome, vertigo, anosmia, tic, frontal sinusitis. Both BL-2 Points (BL-2 on the left and BL-2 on the right) combined with the Extra Point Yin Tang (EX-HN-3) form the "ventral magic triangle." These three points combined have a strong effect on the nasal pharynx (see also EX-HN-3 (p. 130)).

Action in TCM:
- Eliminates Wind
- Clears Heat

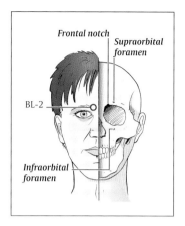

▶ **Fig. 8.4** BL-2.

BL-10 Tian Zhu

"Celestial Pillar" ("Celestial Pillar")

Location: Vertical orientation: 1.3 Cun lateral to the median line (Governing Vessel), in the belly of the trapezius muscle (just at the point where it begins to descend). Point BL-10 is located 0.5 Cun cranial to the dorsal hairline, lateral to GV-15, close to the exit of the greater occipital nerve (▶ **Fig. 8.5**).

Horizontal orientation: above the spinous process of C2 (axis).

> 🛑 **Note**
> BL-10 is located at the level between C1 (atlas) and C2 (axis). On palpation, this region is located cranial to the first palpable vertebral spinous process (since the atlas does not have a spinous process). Palpation is usually easier when the head is slightly retroflexed to relax the nuchal ligament, which is often very tight.

> 🔄 **Practical Tip**
> BL-10 is located slightly more medial and caudal than GB-20 (p. 104).

Depth of needling: 0.5 to 1 Cun, perpendicularly.

> 🔄 **Practical Tip**
> To eliminate any possibility of puncturing the spinal cord, especially in cachectic patients, depth of needling should not exceed 1.5 Cun.

Indication: Strong effect on nose and eyes, enhances effect on BL-2 (front–back coupling), generalized vagus effect; anosmia, cervical syndrome, vertigo, migraine, colds, tonsillitis; affects the regulation of the body's overall tone (see GB-20 (p. 104)).

Action in TCM:
- Eliminates Wind
- Clears the head and the sensory openings

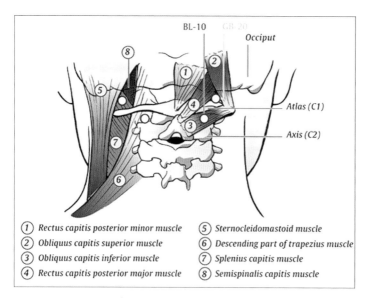

Fig. 8.5 BL-10.

BL-11 Da Zhu

"Great Shuttle" ("Great Axle"), Master Point of the Bones

Location: 1.5 Cun lateral to the lower edge of the spinous process of T1 (▶ **Fig. 8.6**).

❗ Note
With arms hanging down, the distance between the median line and medial margin of the scapula (at the level of the clearly palpable attachment of the scapular spine at the medial margin of the scapula) is 3 Cun.

To make learning easier: The last digit in the numbering of Bladder Channel Points BL-11 to BL-17 follows the numbering of the thoracic vertebrae (e.g., Point BL-11 lies below T1, Point BL-13 below T3).

Depth of needling: 0.5 Cun, perpendicularly or in an oblique medial direction.

> **📝 Practical Tip**
> When needling in an oblique medial direction, guide tip of the needle in a slightly caudal direction.

Indication: Cervical syndrome, shoulder–arm syndrome, sinusitis, effect on "bone disorders," cephalgia, bronchial asthma, feverish colds.

Action in TCM:
- Removes obstructions from the channel
- Relieves pain
- BL-11 (on both sides) + GV-14: The "dorsal magic triangle" has a relaxing and calming effect

BL-13 Fei Shu

"Lung Transport" ("Lung Shu"), Back Shu Point of the Lung

Location: 1.5 Cun lateral to the lower edge of the spinous process of T3 (▶ **Fig. 8.6**).

❗ Note
In standing patients with arms hanging down, the lower edge of the spinous process of T3 is usually located at the level of the attachment of the clearly palpable scapular spine at the medial margin of the scapula.

> **ℹ Additional Information**
> The numbering of the second digit of BL-11 to BL-17 on the Bladder Channel correlates with the numbering of the thoracic vertebrae (e.g., BL-11 is below T1, BL-13 is below T3).

Since the back transport points are segmentally assigned to the organs of the functional circles, the back transport points of the thoracic organs (lungs, circulatory system, heart) lie in the thoracic region, those of the digestive organs (liver, spleen, pancreas, stomach) in the abdominal region, and those of the urogenital organs (kidney, bladder) in the lumbar region.

Depth of needling: 0.5 Cun, perpendicularly or obliquely.

> **Practical Tip**
> When needling in an oblique medial direction, guide the needle slightly in a caudal direction to avoid any possibility of puncturing the spinal cord.

Indication: Respiratory tract disorders, asthma, cough, dyspnea, night sweats.

Action in TCM:
- Distributes and regulates Lung Qi
- Supports the descending functions of the Lung

BL-14 Jue Yin Shu

"Jue Yin Back Transport Point" ("Pericardium Shu"), Back Shu Point of the Pericardium

Location: 1.5 Cun lateral to the lower edge of the spinous process of T4 (▶ **Fig. 8.6**).

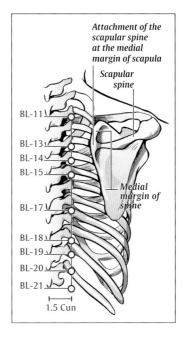

Attachment of the scapular spine at the medial margin of scapula

Scapular spine

BL-11
BL-13
BL-14
BL-15

Medial margin of spine

BL-17
BL-18
BL-19
BL-20
BL-21

1.5 Cun

▶ **Fig. 8.6** BL-11, BL-13, and BL-14.

Depth of needling: 0.5 Cun, perpendicularly or in an oblique medial–caudal direction (see BL-11 (p. 68) and BL-13 (p. 68)).

Indication: Functional heart problems, singultus (hiccup), psychosomatic problems, angina pectoris, bronchitis, bronchial asthma, circulatory dysregulation.

Action in TCM: Regulates the Heart.

BL-15 Xin Shu

"Heart Transport" ("Heart Shu"), Back Shu Point of the Heart

Location: 1.5 Cun lateral to the lower edge of the spinous process of T5 (▶ **Fig. 8.7**).

Depth of needling: 0.5 Cun, perpendicularly or in an oblique medial–caudal direction (see BL-11 (p.68) and BL-13 (p.68)).

Indication: "Heart disorders," fever, night sweats, menopause problems, insomnia, restlessness.

Action in TCM:
- Tonifies the Brain and nourishes the Heart
- Sedates or calms the Mind (Shen)

BL-17 Ge Shu

"Diaphragm Transport" ("Diaphragm Shu"), Back Shu Point of the Diaphragm, Master Point of the Blood

Location: 1.5 Cun lateral to the lower edge of the spinous process of T7 (▶ **Fig. 8.7**).

Depth of needling: 0.5 Cun, perpendicularly or in an oblique medial–caudal direction (see BL-11 (p.68) and BL-13 (p.68)).

Indication: Pronounced effect on the diaphragm; singultus (hiccup), vomiting, bronchial asthma, hematological disorders with a "venous component," dyspnea, urticaria.

Action in TCM:
- Regulates Blood
- Clears Blood Heat
- Removes Blood Stagnation

🛈 Note

In standing patients with arms hanging down, the lower edge of T7 is usually located at the level of the inferior angle of the scapula.

ℹ Additional Information

The numbering of the second digit of BL-11 to BL-17 on the Bladder Channel correlates with the numbering of the thoracic vertebrae (e.g., BL-11 is below T1, BL-13 is below T3).

BL-18 Gan Shu

"Liver Transport" ("Liver Shu"),
Back Shu Point of the Liver

Location: 1.5 Cun lateral to the lower edge of the spinous process of T9 (▶ **Fig. 8.7**).

ℹ **Additional Information**
Up to BL-17, the last digit in the numbering of Bladder Channel Points corresponds to the numbering of the thoracic vertebrae (e.g., BL-17 is located below T7). Starting with BL-18, one vertebra is added (e.g., BL-18 is located below T9).

Depth of needling: 0.5 Cun, perpendicularly or in an oblique medial–caudal direction (see BL-11 (p. 68) and BL-13 (p. 68)).

Indication: Liver metabolism disorders, vision disorders, vertigo, tension in the epigastric and hypochondriac region, menstruation cycle disorders, muscle tension, muscle cramps, pain in the upper abdomen, emotional hyperexcitability.

Action in TCM: Regulates Liver Qi.

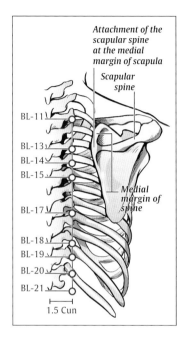

▶ **Fig. 8.7** BL-15, BL-17, and BL-18.

BL-19 Dan Shu

"Gallbladder Transport" ("Gallbladder Shu"), Back Shu Point of the Gallbladder

Location: 1.5 Cun lateral to the lower edge of the spinous process of T10 (▶ **Fig. 8.8**).

Depth of needling: 0.5 Cun, perpendicularly or in an oblique medial-caudal direction (see BL-11 (p.68) and BL-13 (p.68)).

Indication: Gallbladder disorders, vomiting, bitter taste in the mouth, acid reflux.

Action in TCM: Regulates Liver and Gallbladder.

BL-20 Pi Shu

"Spleen Transport" ("Spleen Shu"), Back Shu Point of the Spleen

Location: 1.5 Cun lateral to the lower edge of the spinous process of T11 (▶ **Fig. 8.8**).

Depth of needling: 0.5 Cun, perpendicularly or in an oblique medial–caudal direction (see BL-11 (p.68) and BL-13 (p.68)).

Indication: Important point for treating the gastrointestinal tract; meteorism, dysentery, loss of appetite, stomach and duodenal ulcers, abdominal sensation of tension and fullness, diarrhea, edematous swellings, chronic mucus disorders of the respiratory tract, convalescence.

Action in TCM:
- Tonifies and nourishes:
  - Spleen Qi and Spleen Yang
  - Blood

BL-21 Wei Shu

"Stomach Transport," "Stomach Shu," Back Shu Point of the Stomach

Location: 1.5 Cun lateral to the lower edge of the spinous process of T12 (▶ **Fig. 8.8**).

Depth of needling: 0.5 Cun, perpendicularly or in an oblique medial–caudal direction.

Indication: Stomach disorders, digestive problems, nausea, vomiting, gastric motility disorders, singultus (hiccup), loss of appetite.

Action in TCM: Regulates and descends Stomach Qi.

BL-23 Shen Shu

"Kidney Transport" ("Kidney Shu," "Sea of Vitality"), Back Shu Point of the Kidney

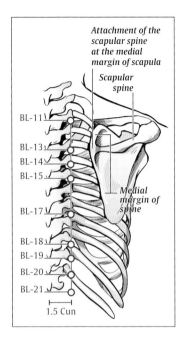

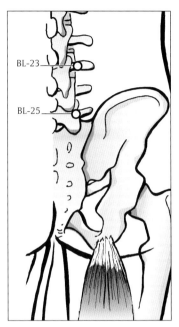

▶ **Fig. 8.8** BL-19, BL-20, and BL-21.

▶ **Fig. 8.9** BL-23.

Location: 1.5 Cun lateral to the lower edge of the spinous process of L2 (▶ **Fig. 8.9**).

Note

To locate vertebra L2, it is recommended to start at the iliac crest (vertebra L4, see BL-25 (p. 74)).

Depth of needling: 0.5 to 1.5 Cun, perpendicularly.

Indication: Excellent point for strengthening renal function and renal circulation, for all chronic disorders: chronic weakness and exhaustion, chronic lumbago, chronic asthma, urogenital tract disorders, allergies, rheumatic disorders. This point is one of the very important points often used with moxa.

J. Bischko: For conditions that worsen with cold temperatures.

Action in TCM:
- Tonifies and nourishes:
  - Kidney
  - Kidney Yang and supports Essence (Jing)
- Regulates water balance and promotes diuresis
- Strengthens lower back, ears, eyes, and uterus

BL-25 Da Chang Shu

**"Large Intestine Transport"
("Large Intestine Shu"), Back Shu
Point of the Large Intestine**

Location: 1.5 Cun lateral to the
lower edge of the spinous process
of L4 (▶ **Fig. 8.10**).

❗ Note
Vertebra L4 is located at the level
of the iliac crest (palpation from
caudal to prevent skin folds from
being pressed onto the iliac
crest). The lower edge of the spinous process lies a bit deeper.

Depth of needling: 0.5 to 1.5
Cun, perpendicularly.

Indication: Obstipation, diarrhea,
disorders of the large intestine;
important local point in cases of
lumbago.

Action in TCM:
* Supports and regulates intesti-
  nal function
* Loosens Stagnation and relieves
  pain

BL-27 Xiao Chang Shu

**"Small Intestine Transport"
("Small Intestine Shu"), Back Shu
Point of the Small Intestine**

Location: At the level of the first
sacral foramen, 1.5 Cun lateral to
the dorsal median line, in a

depression between the sacrum
and the upper region of the posterior superior iliac spine (▶ **Fig. 8.11**).

❗ Note
On palpation of the posterior
superior iliac spine, BL-27 is
located in a cranial and medial
direction. Palpation of the posterior superior iliac spine is always
performed from caudal because
the bony pole is curved caudally.

Aid in localizing the posterior
superior iliac spine: Starting at the
intergluteal (anal) cleft, palpate
approximately 3 Cun at an angle
of 45° in a laterocranial direction.

Depth of needling: 0.5 to 1.5
Cun, perpendicularly; possibly in
a slightly oblique lateral direction
toward the sacroiliac joint.

Indication: Lumbago, genital disorders, spontaneous ejaculation,
enuresis.

Action in TCM: Regulates
intestines and bladder.

BL-28 Pang Guang Shu

**"Bladder Transport" ("Bladder
Shu"), Back Shu Point of the
Bladder**

Location: At the level of the
second sacral foramen, 1.5 Cun
lateral to the dorsal median line.
On palpation of the posterior

superior iliac spine (see BL-27 (p. 74)), BL-28 is located slightly caudal and medial (▶ Fig. 8.11).

Depth of needling: 0.5 to 1.5 Cun, perpendicularly; possibly in a slightly oblique lateral direction toward the sacroiliac joint.

Indication: Lumbago, bladder disorders.

Action in TCM:
- Regulates bladder
- Clears Heat

BL-36 Cheng Fu

"Support" ("Supporting by Hand")

Location: In the middle of the gluteal (anal) crease (not of the thigh) (▶ Fig. 8.11).

🔋 Functional Note
This point is located in close proximity to the sciatic nerve. With deep needling, it is possible to puncture the nerve. The needle's position in the perineural tissue explains part of the acupuncture effect.

Depth of needling: 0.5 to 1.5 Cun, perpendicularly.

Indication: Lumbago–sciatica.

🔋 Note
BL-36 is located over the ischial tuberosity. This point is also

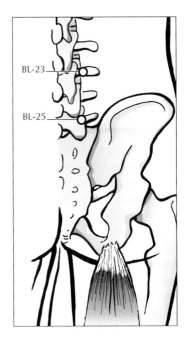

▶ **Fig. 8.10** BL-25.

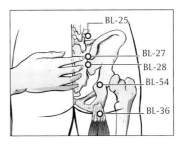

▶ **Fig. 8.11** BL-27, BL-28, and BL-36.

painful in enthesopathy of the ischiocrural muscles (semitendinous muscle, semimembranous muscle, biceps muscle of the thigh).

Action in TCM: Removes obstructions in the channel.

BL-40 Wei Zhong

"Bend Center" ("Popliteal Center"), Lower Sea Point (Lower He Point) of the Bladder

Location: In the middle of the popliteal cavity. This point lies close to the tibial nerve and the popliteal artery (▸ **Fig. 8.12**).

Depth of needling: 0.5 to 1 Cun, perpendicularly.

Indication: Lumbago, gonalgia, paresis of the lower extremity; important distant point for the lower lumbar spine region; skin disorders, kidney and bladder disorders, eczema, herpes zoster, psoriasis (Blood Heat, microphlebotomy), dysuria.
   H. Schmidt: Microphlebotomy is often a good idea.

Action in TCM:
- Regulates flow of Qi in the lower lumbar spine and loosens Stagnation
- Supports the bladder
- Cools Blood Heat

> **Practical Tip**
> Use BL-40 for conditions of repletion; BL-60 is better suited for chronic conditions (vacuity) and symptoms of Cold.

BL-43 Gao Huang

"Gao Huang Transport" ("Vital Organs")

Location: 3 Cun lateral to the lower edge of the spinous process of T4 (▸ **Fig. 8.13**).

> **Note**
> The localization of BL-43 corresponds to a very frequent trigger point in the greater rhomboid muscle or in the iliocostal muscle of the thorax. With deep needling, the tip of the needle passes through quite a few muscles (ascending part of trapezius muscle, greater rhomboid muscle, iliocostal muscle of the thorax), which are innervated by the spinal nerves of various segments (C4–C5, T1–T4). The ascending part of the trapezius muscle developed embryologically from portions of the head mesenchyme and is innervated by the accessory nerve. This explains the broad effect of BL-43, covering several segments. Further indications, see below.

Depth of needling: 0.5 to 1 Cun, subcutaneously in an oblique direction toward BL-14 (enhancing the effect), or 0.5 Cun in a

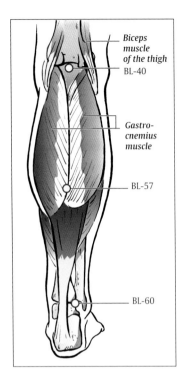

▶ **Fig. 8.12** BL-40.

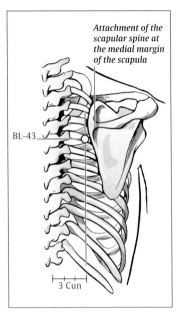

▶ **Fig. 8.13** BL-43.

vertical direction, using the two-finger-protection method.

Indication: Respiratory tract disorders, sleep disorders, palpitations, concentration problems, erectile dysfunction, gastrointestinal disorders, back pain; broad spectrum of indications: this point is indicated in chronic disorders that are otherwise resistant to therapy.

Action in TCM:
- Tonifies and nourishes:
  - Lung, Heart, Kidney, Spleen, and Stomach
  - Blood and Yin
- Clears Vacuity Heat
- Supports Essence (Jing)
- Calms and supports the Mind (Shen)

BL-54 Zhi Bian

"Sequential Limit" ("Lowermost in Order")

Location: 3 Cun lateral to the sacral hiatus, at the level of the fourth sacral foramen (▶ Fig. 8.14).

❗ Note

Needling of BL-54 first reaches the gluteus maximus muscle and, still deeper, the piriformis muscle. There are important trigger points of both these muscles in this location. Tensions in both muscles play a major role in causing pain in the lumbar–pelvic–hip region. Since the sciatic nerve is located in the depth, there is a risk of puncturing it by deep needling. In about 20% of cases, the sciatic nerve runs through the piriformis muscle. This is also the case when the point of ramification is high; the fibular part runs through the piriformis muscle while the tibial part runs through the infrapiriform foramen. This explains the irritation and pain that can result when the tone of the piriformis muscle increases; hence, painfulness is not always the only cause of trigger points in this region.

Depth of needling: Very deep, sometimes up to 4 Cun.

Indication: Important distant point for lumbar spine problems (use deep needling); segmental relationship.

Action in TCM: Removes obstructions in the channel and relieves pain.

BL-57 Cheng Shan

"Mountain Support" ("Supporting Hill")

Location: Halfway between BL-40 and BL-60; 8 Cun caudal to BL-40, in a depression between the bellies of the gastrocnemius muscle (▶ Fig. 8.15).

❗ Note

Standing on the toes clearly demonstrates the calf muscles (especially the gastrocnemius muscle).

Another way of localization is by means of the hand span method: in the middle between BL-40 and BL-60 (see also ST-38 (p. 42)).

Depth of needling: 0.5 to 1 Cun, perpendicularly.

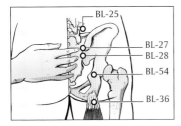

▶ **Fig. 8.14** BL-54.

Indication: Sciatica-like problems, cramps in the calf muscles, pain in the Achilles tendon; important distant point for lumbar spine problems and for the anal region (hemorrhoids), peripheral circulation disorders (intermittent claudication).

Action in TCM: Removes obstructions in the channel.

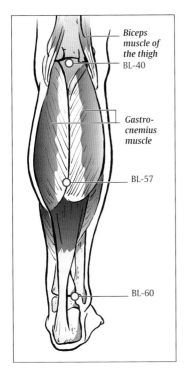

▶ **Fig. 8.15** BL-57.

BL-60 Kun Lun

"Kunlun Mountains" ("Big and High")

Location: In the middle of the line connecting the lateral malleolus and Achilles tendon (▶ **Fig. 8.16**).

❗ Note
The De Qi sensation often appears strongly when the needle is directed toward the calcaneus. BL-60 is often described in the literature as lying opposite KI-3. However, this is not the case, because the outer and inner ankle bones do not lie on the same level.

Depth of needling: 0.5 to 1 Cun, perpendicularly.

Indication: One of the major peripheral pain points, especially for the lower extremity.
    Pain syndromes of the spine, cephalgia, pain in the Achilles tendon, disorders in the region of the ankle joint; painful menstruation during dysmenorrhea, with dark, clotted menstrual blood; protracted course of childbirth, placental retention.

Action in TCM:
- Supports the spine
- Removes Blood Stagnation

❗ Note
Do not perform sedating stimulation during pregnancy.

BL-62 Shen Mai

"Extending Vessel" ("Stretching Channel"), Opening Point of the Extraordinary Channel, Yang Qiao Mai (Yang Heel Vessel)

Location: In a depression, directly below the tip of the lateral malleolus, in the articular cavity between the talus and calcaneus (▶ **Fig. 8.16**).

ℹ Additional Information
In the Chinese literature this point is sometimes localized directly caudal to the lateral malleolus. This makes it a good idea to localize this point by searching for the maximum pain frequency (*Very Point Method* according to Gleditsch).

Depth of needling: 3 to 5 mm, perpendicularly.

Indication: Tension headache, psychovegetative dysregulation, peroneal neuralgia and paresis, dysfunction of the talocalcaneal joints (pronation, supination).
    Proven combination: SI-3 + BL-62 for tension headache.

H. Schmidt: Pain in the inner corner of the eye.

Action in TCM:

- Removes obstructions in the channel
- Relaxes tendons and muscles
- Relieves pain

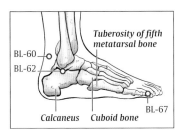

▶ **Fig. 8.16** BL-60, BL-62 and BL-67.

BL-67 Zhi Yin

"Reaching Yin" ("Reaching Inside"), Tonification Point

Location: Lateral corner of the nail of the fifth toe (▶ **Fig. 8.16**).

Depth of needling: 1 to 2 mm, perpendicularly; let it bleed if necessary.

Indication: Cephalgia, urinary retention, uterine inertia; facilitating labor, correcting fetal malposition (moxa).

🔳 Note
Do not perform downward (descending) stimulation during pregnancy.

Action in TCM:

- Expels Wind
- Clears the Mind (Shen) and the eyes

9 Kidney Channel

▶ Fig. 9.1, ▶ Fig. 9.2

Major Points

- KI-3: Source point (Yuan Point)
- KI-6: Opening point of the extraordinary channel, Yin Qiao Mai (Yin Heel Vessel)
- KI-7: Tonification point
- KI-27: Local point

Associated Points

- GB-25: Front collecting point (Mu Point) of the kidney
- BL-23: Back transport point (Back Shu Point) of the kidney

Coupling Relationships

▶ Fig. 9.3

Top-to-bottom coupling:
Heart–kidney

Yin-Yang coupling: Kidney–bladder

KI-3 Tai Xi

"Great Ravine" ("Big Stream"), Source Point (Yuan Point)

Location: In the middle of the line connecting the greatest prominence of the medial malleolus with the Achilles tendon (▶ **Fig. 9.4**).

Depth of needling: 0.5 to 1 Cun, perpendicularly.

Indication: Excellent point for strengthening renal function and circulation; psychovegetative exhaustion, erectile dysfunction, enuresis, painful menstruation, urogenital tract disorders, pain in the Achilles tendon, disorders of the ankle joints.

Action in TCM:
- Tonifies and nourishes:
  - Kidney Qi
  - Kidney Yang
  - Kidney Yin

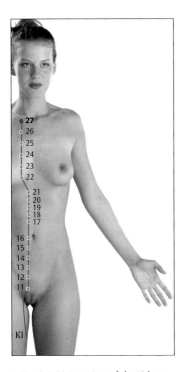

▶ **Fig. 9.1** Major points of the Kidney Channel (1).

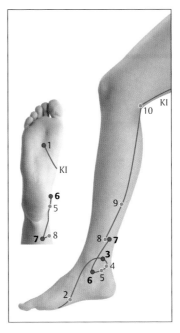

▶ **Fig. 9.2** Major points of the Kidney Channel (2).

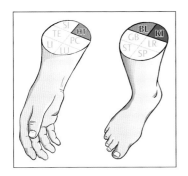

▶ **Fig. 9.3** Coupling relationships of the Kidney Channel.

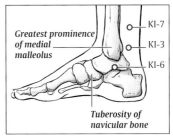

▶ **Fig. 9.4** KI-3.

KI-6 Zhao Hai

"Shining Sea" ("Shine on Sea"), Opening Point of the Extraordinary Channel, Yin Qiao Mai (Yin Heel Vessel)

Location: 0.5 Cun caudal to the medial malleolus, in the region of the articular cavity between the talus and calcaneus, in the region of the sustentaculum of talus (▶ Fig. 9.5).

KI-6 is located at the same level as BL-62.

! Note

The tibiocalcaneal part of the deltoid ligament expands between the medial malleolus and sustentaculum of the talus of the calcaneus. This ligament is important for stabilizing the inner malleolus. Many proprioceptors are located here, near the talocalcaneal joint. The importance of talocalcaneal joint function for complete, balanced human motion is also known to chiropractic.

KI-6 is the Opening Point for the Extraordinary Channel, Yin Qiao Mai. The translation of Qiao is "heel" (of the dancing girl), "mobility." Both Yin Qiao Mai and Yang Qiao Mai balance the Yang and Yin muscle tone, regulate mobility of the joints, and affect the Bi syndrome (rheumatic symptoms).

Depth of needling: 0.3 to 0.5 Cun, perpendicularly.

Indication: Urogenital tract disorders; balancing effect on hormonal disorders, migraine, sleep disorders, night sweats, itching of the external genitals; general symptoms of chronic dryness (especially of the eyes); dry mucosa in the throat area, dry skin, dysfunction of the upper ankle joint and talocalcaneal joint.

J. Bischko: A major point for mental and emotional tonification.

Action in TCM:
- Tonifies and nourishes:
  - Kidney Functional Circle
  - Kidney Yin

KI-7 Fu Liu

"Recover Flow" ("Continuing Stream"), Tonification Point

Location: 2 Cun above KI-3, at the anterior margin of the Achilles tendon (▶ Fig. 9.5).

Depth of needling: 0.5 to 1 Cun, perpendicularly.

Indication: Important point for urogenital disorders, chronic lumbago and gonalgia, lack of motivation, depression, mental and physical exhaustion, morning diarrhea.

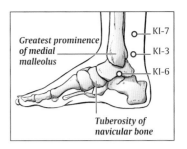

▶ **Fig. 9.5** KI-6 and KI-7.

Action in TCM:
- Tonifies and nourishes:
  - Kidney Functional Circle
  - Kidney Qi and Kidney Yang

KI-27 Shu Fu

"Transport Mansion" ("Shu Mansion")

Location: Right under the clavicle, 2 Cun lateral to the median line, in close proximity to the sternoclavicular joint (▶ **Fig. 9.6**).

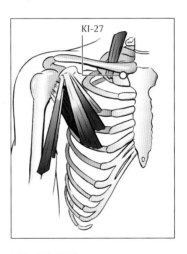

▶ **Fig. 9.6** KI-27.

Depth of needling: 2 to 4 mm, perpendicularly.

> Caution
> Deep needling carries the risk of pneumothorax.

Indication: Important point for treating asthma, chest pain.

Action in TCM: Relaxes the thorax.

10 Pericardium Channel

▶ Fig. 10.1

Major Points

- PC-3: Local point
- PC-6: Connecting point (Luo Point). Opening point of the Extraordinary Channel, Yin Wei Mai (Yin Linking Vessel)
- PC-7: Source point (Yuan Point), sedation point

Associated Points

- CV-17: Front collecting point (Mu Point) of the pericardium
- BL-14: Back transport point (Back Shu Point) of the pericardium

Coupling Relationships

▶ Fig. 10.2

Top-to-bottom coupling: Pericardium–liver
Yin-Yang coupling: Pericardium–Triple Energizer

PC-3 Qu Ze

"Marsh at the Bend" ("Crooked Marsh")

Location: Ulnar to the biceps tendon, in the crease of the elbow (▶ Fig. 10.3).

Depth of needling: 0.5 to 1 Cun, perpendicularly.

Indication: Epicondylopathia, angina pectoris, tachycardia, restlessness and panic attacks, fever and skin rashes, hypermenorrhea.

Action in TCM:
- Clears Heat
- Calms the Mind (Shen)

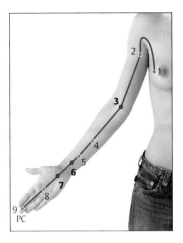

▶ **Fig. 10.1** Major points of the Pericardium Channel.

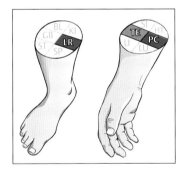

▶ **Fig. 10.2** Coupling relationships of the Pericardium Channel.

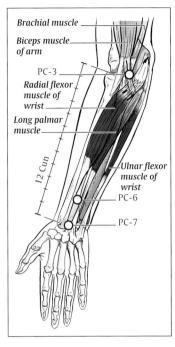

Brachial muscle

Biceps muscle of arm

PC-3

Radial flexor muscle of wrist

Long palmar muscle

12 Cun

Ulnar flexor muscle of wrist

PC-6

PC-7

▶ **Fig. 10.3** PC-3, PC-6, and PC-7.

PC-6 Nei Guan

"Inner Pass" ("Inner Pass"), Connecting Point (Luo Point), Opening Point of the Extraordinary Channel, Yin Wei Mai (Yin Linking Vessel)

Location: 2 Cun proximal to the crease of the wrist, between the tendons of the long palmar muscle and the radial flexor muscle of the wrist (▶ **Fig. 10.4**).

As described for localizing HT-7, use the wrist crease that is located between the radius and ulna and the proximal carpal bones. The proximal carpal bones are marked by the pisiform bone. The crease in question is located proximal to pisiform bone.

🄸 Note

To localize this point precisely, the "dynamic palpation" technique described for TE-5 is recommended. Shifting the skin fold palmar between the radial flexor muscle of the wrist and the long palmar muscle in a proximal direction creates a thickening of the skin fold, which "catches" at PC-6. PC-6 is located opposite TE-5.

Depth of needling: 0.5 Cun, perpendicularly.

Indication: Important functional point, pre-eminent acupuncture point for pain and disorders in the thoracic and epigastric regions; strong mental and emotional balancing effect, especially for states of anxiety and agitation; functional heart problems, nausea, vomiting, singultus (hiccup).

Action in TCM:
- Regulates Heart Qi and Heart Blood and sedates and/or calms the Mind (Shen)
- Descends rebellious Lung Qi and Stomach Qi

PC-7 Da Ling

"Great Mound" ("Big Mound"), Source Point (Yuan Point), Sedation Point

Location: In the middle of the wrist crease, between the tendons of the long palmar muscle and the radial flexor muscle of the wrist (▶ **Fig. 10.4**).

(For help in localizing the wrist crease, see HT-7 (p. 52)).

Depth of needling: 0.3 to 0.5 Cun, perpendicularly.

Indication: Disorders in the wrist region, enthesopathy in the lower arm region, functional heart problems, emotional states of agitation and anxiety.

J. Bischko: Strong analgesic effect for herpes zoster, writer's cramp.

Action in TCM:
- Regulates the Heart
- Clears the Mind (Shen)

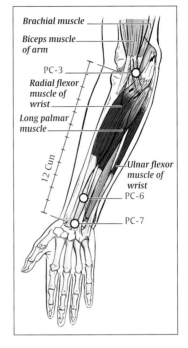

▶ **Fig. 10.4** PC-3, PC-6, and PC-7.

11 Triple Energizer Channel

San Jiao Channel known as Triple Energizer (TE, 3E) Channel, but also as Triple Warmer, Triple Burner (TB) or Triple Heater (TH).

▶ Fig. 11.1

Major Points

- TE-3: Tonification point
- TE-4: Source point (Yuan Point)
- TE-5: Connecting point (Luo Point). Opening point of the extraordinary channel, Yang Wei Mai (Yang Linking Vessel)
- TE-14: Local point
- TE-15: Local point
- TE-17: Local point
- TE-21: Local point

Associated Points

- CV-5: Front collecting point (Mu Point) of the Triple Energizer
- BL-22: Back transport point (Back Shu Point) of the Triple Energizer
- BL-39: Lower sea point (Lower He Point) of the Triple Energizer

Coupling Relationships

▶ Fig. 11.2

Top-to-bottom coupling: Triple Energizer–gallbladder
Yang-Yin coupling: Triple Energizer–pericardium

TE-3 Zhong Zhu

"Central Islet," Tonification Point

Location: In a depression on the back of the hand, between fourth and fifth metacarpal bones, close to their body–head transition (▶ Fig. 11.3).

Depth of needling: 0.5 to 1 Cun, obliquely in a proximal direction.

Indication: Important point for ear disorders, tinnitus, hearing loss, vertigo, cephalgia, pain and paresis in the upper extremity.

Action in TCM:
- Eliminates Wind
- Clears Heat

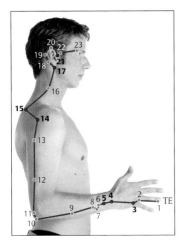

▶ **Fig. 11.1** Major points of the Triple Energizer Channel.

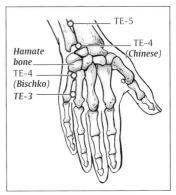

▶ **Fig. 11.3** TE-3.

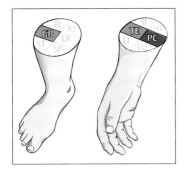

▶ **Fig. 11.2** Coupling relationships of the Triple Energizer Channel.

TE-4 Yang Chi

**"Yang Pool" ("Active Pond"),
Source Point (Yuan Point)**

Location: Slightly ulnar to the middle of the dorsal wrist crease (articular cavity between radius–ulna and proximal carpal bones), ulnar to the tendon of the extensor muscle of the fingers, radial to the tendon of the extensor muscle of the little finger (▶ Fig. 11.4).

❗ Note
The easiest way to find the tendon of the extensor muscle of the fingers is by moving the second, third and fourth fingers as though playing on a keyboard. The dorsal wrist crease often becomes visible only upon dorsal flexion of the hand. If the tendon still remains indistinct, orient yourself on a slightly convex, bow-shaped line running in a proximal direction between the styloid processes of the radius and ulna.

According to J. Bischko, TE-4 is localized further distal, at the level of the articular cavity between the fourth and fifth metacarpal bones and the hamate bone. This point is often much more sensitive to pressure than the point localized according to the Chinese method. When in doubt, the deciding factor is pressure sensitivity.

Depth of needling: Approx. 0.3 Cun, perpendicularly.

Indication: Wrist disorders, pain and paresis in the upper extremity.
  H. Schmidt: Moxibustion of TE-4 on the left hand has a general stimulating effect, especially on the organs of the lower abdomen.
  J. Bischko: Master point for cluster (vasomotor) headache.

Action in TCM: Removes obstructions in the channel.

TE-5 Wai Guan

"Outer Pass," Connecting Point (Luo Point), Opening Point of the Extraordinary Channel Yang Wei Mai (Yang Linking Vessel)

Location: 2 Cun proximal to TE-4 (p. 92) (slightly ulnar to the middle of the dorsal wrist crease; see TE-4 (p. 92)), on a line connecting TE-4 with the tip of the olecranon (▶ Fig. 11.4).

📋 Practical Tip
TE-4 is localized on the lower arm, between radius and ulna, on a line connecting TE-5 and the end of the olecranon. With the lower arm in supination (as shown in the dorsal view in ▶ Fig. 11.4), the connecting line is located approximately in the middle of the extensor muscle side of the lower arm.

Normally, however, with patients lying on their back, the lower arms are in pronation. When that is the case, the connecting line runs distinctly ulnar to the median line toward the olecranon.

In this arm position, the line between TE-4 and the head of the radius is used for orientation. TE-5 is located directly ulnar to this orientation line.

Note

TE-5 can be located more quickly using dynamic palpation. Slide the examining index finger from the dorsal wrist crease in a proximal direction between the radius and ulna. At TE-5, the finger feels a distinct "catch" as the skin fold

thickness increases. TE-5 is located almost opposite PC-6.

Depth of needling: 0.5 to 1 Cun, perpendicularly or in an oblique proximal direction.

Indication: Cephalgia, cervical syndrome, tinnitus, wrist disorders, hearing loss; major point for sensitivity to changes in the weather; pain and paresis in the upper extremity, feverish colds, skin eczema.

J. Bischko: Master point for rheumatic disorders.

Action in TCM:
- Eliminates Wind
- Clears Heat

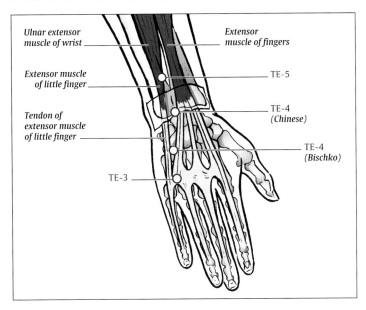

Ulnar extensor muscle of wrist

Extensor muscle of fingers

Extensor muscle of little finger

TE-5

TE-4 (Chinese)

Tendon of extensor muscle of little finger

TE-4 (Bischko)

TE-3

▶ **Fig. 11.4** TE-4 (Bischko), TE-4 (Chinese), and TE-5.

TE-14 Jian Liao

"Shoulder Bone-Hole"

Location: In "the posterior shoulder depression" which forms when the arm is abducted 90°, slightly caudal to the dorsal pole of the acromion (▶ **Fig. 11.5**).

Depth of needling: 0.5 to 1.5 Cun, perpendicularly or in an oblique distal direction.

🛈 Note

TE-14 is located where the acromial part and the spinal part of the deltoid muscle come together at the dorsal acromion pole. In muscular persons, the different components of the deltoid muscle (clavicular, acromial, and spinal parts) are prominent and the muscle grooves are easy to follow. TE-14 is located at the cranial end of the posterior groove, caudal to the dorsal pole of the acromion. The dorsal pole of the acromion can be located by following the course of the easily palpable scapular spine in a lateral direction.

Indication: Pain in the shoulder region; important local point.

Action in TCM: Removes obstructions in the channel.

TE-15 Tian Liao

"Celestial Bone-Hole" ("Celestial Crevice")

Location: 1 Cun caudal to Point GB-21, midway between GB-21 and SI-13, on the superior angle of the scapula (▶ **Fig. 11.6**).

(Localizing GB-21: Midway between the lower edge of the spinous process of C7 and the acromion.

Localizing SI-13: Midway between the lower edge of the spinous process of T2 and SI-10 (▶ **Fig. 7.6**), in the elongation of the dorsal fold of the arm pit, right above the scapular spine.)

Depth of needling: 0.5 to 0.8 Cun, perpendicularly.

⎯ Caution ⎯⎯⎯⎯⎯⎯⎯
Risk of pneumothorax.

🛈 Note

For information about localization of C7, see GB-21 (p. 106)

Indication: Cephalgia, cervical syndrome, torticollis, sensitivity to changes in the weather.
J. Bischko: Master point for the arms.

Action in TCM: Removes obstructions in the channel.

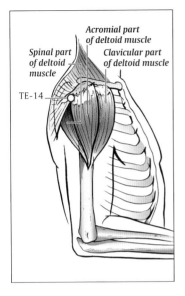

▶ **Fig. 11.5** TE-14.

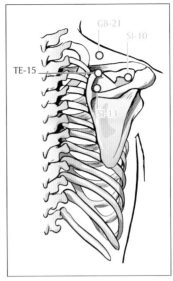

▶ **Fig. 11.6** TE-15.

TE-17 Yi Feng

"Wind Screen" ("Shielding Wind")

Location: Behind the ear lobe, between the mandible and mastoid process (▶ Fig. 11.7).

> **⚡ Practical Tip**
> TE-17 is located in close proximity to the facial nerve, which exits here from the stylomastoid foramen. Therefore, there is a risk of puncturing this nerve when needling deeply.

Depth of needling: 0.5 to 1.5 Cun, perpendicularly or obliquely toward the front.

> **❗ Note**
> The tip of the needle ends up positioned very close to the transverse process of the atlas, which can usually be palpated easily between the mandible and the mastoid process. This explains the point's effect on the upper head joints (see Indication below (p. 96)). In addition, this location is close to the vertebral artery. That's why this point is needled from the front.

Indication: Tinnitus, hearing loss, cephalgia, trigeminal neuralgia, facial neuralgia, facial paresis, spasmolysis.

The upper head joints (atlanto-occipital joints) influence the overall tone of the body and play an important role as a peripheral balancing organ.

Action in TCM:
- Eliminates Wind
- Clears Heat

TE-21 Er Men

"Ear Gate" ("Ear Door")

Location: At the level of the supratragic notch above SI-19, immediately behind the upper dorsal portion of the condylar process of the mandible (▶ Fig. 11.7, ▶ Fig. 11.8).

Depth of needling: 0.5 Cun, perpendicularly or subcutaneously in a caudal direction.

> **❗ Note**
> Insert the needle with the patient's mouth slightly opened. This causes the temporomandibular joint to move slightly in a ventral direction and prevents the risk of injury to the joint (depth of needling approx. 0.5 Cun). Once the needle is inserted, the patient's mouth is closed. Another possibility is subcutaneous needling in the direction of SI-19 and GB-2.

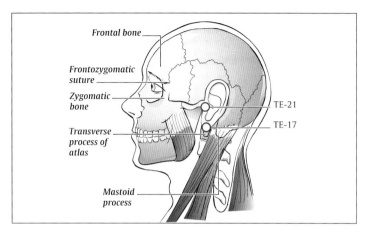

▶ **Fig. 11.7** TE-17.

Moving the needle forward more or less deeply also influences these points and increases the effect of TE-21 (same indications for SI-19 and GB-2 as for TE-21).

✓ Practical Tip
TE-21 is located in very close proximity to the superficial temporal artery. To avoid puncturing this vessel, palpate its pulse prior to needling.

Indication: Ear disorders, gnathologic disorders, toothache, cephalgia.

Action in TCM:
- Supports the ear
- Promotes hearing
- Eliminates Wind

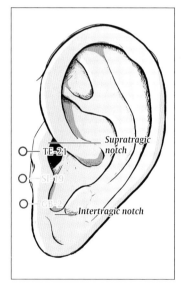

▶ **Fig. 11.8** TE-21.

12   Gallbladder Channel

▶ Fig. 12.1, ▶ Fig. 12.2

Major Points

- GB-2: Local point
- GB-8: Local point
- GB-14: Local point
- GB-20: Point with broad regulatory effect on Wind Disorders
- GB-21: Local point
- GB-30: Local point
- GB-34: Lower sea point (Lower He Point) of the gallbladder. Master point of the muscles and tendons
- GB-39: Master point of the bone marrow
- GB-41: Opening point of the extraordinary channel Dai Mai (Girdle Vessel)

Associated Points

- GB-24: Front collecting point (Mu Point) of the gallbladder
- BL-19: Back transport point (Back Shu Point) of the gallbladder
- GB-34: Lower Sea Point (Lower He Point) of the gallbladder

Coupling Relationships

▶ Fig. 12.3

Top-to-bottom coupling:
Triple Energizer–gallbladder
Yang-Yin coupling: Gallbladder–liver

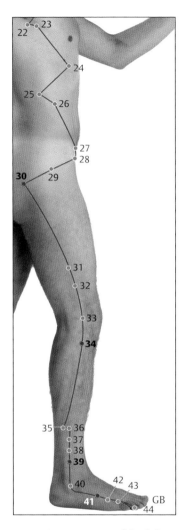

▶ **Fig. 12.1** Major points of the Gall-bladder Channel (1).

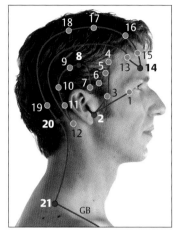

▶ **Fig. 12.2** Major points of the Gall-bladder Channel (2).

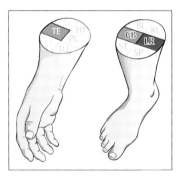

▶ **Fig. 12.3** Coupling relationships of the Gallbladder Channel.

GB-2 Ting Hui

"Auditory Convergence" ("Listening Convergence")

Location: In front of the intertragic notch, directly below SI-19 (depression in front of the tragus when the mouth is slightly opened), in front of the posterior edge of the condylar process of the mandible (mandibular condyle) (► **Fig. 12.4**).

🛑 Note

Insert the needle with the patient's mouth slightly opened. This causes the temporomandibular joint to move slightly in a ventral direction and prevents the risk of injuring the joint (depth of needling, approx. 0.5 Cun). Once the needle is inserted, the patient's mouth is closed.

For ear disorders, TE-21, SI-19, and GB-2 can all be reached together with one needle. For this purpose, the needle is pushed from TE-21 subcutaneously in a caudal direction until GB-2 is reached.

🔁 Practical Tip

GB-2 is located in close proximity to the superficial temporal artery. To avoid puncturing this vessel, palpate its pulse prior to needling.

Depth of needling: 0.5 to 1 Cun, perpendicularly (see also 'Note' above).

Indication: Gnathologic problems, ear disorders, migraine, tinnitus, toothache.

Action in TCM:
- Opens the ear
- Eliminates Wind

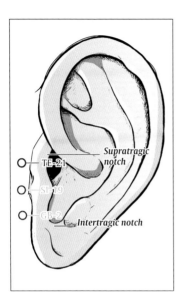

Supratragic
notch

TE-21

SI-19

GB-2

Intertragic notch

▶ **Fig. 12.4** GB-2.

GB-8 Shuai Gu

"Valley Lead" ("Following the Valley")

Location: 1.5 Cun above the highest point of the auricle (▶ **Fig. 12.5**).

Depth of needling: 0.3 to 0.5 Cun, obliquely in the direction of the pain site.

Indication: Parietal and temporal cephalgia.

J. Bischko: Needling of Points GB-8 on both sides of the head and of GV-20 (Du Mai 20) causes horizontal flow through the head. Vertical flow is promoted by needling the following Points: PdM (Point de Merveille; also called Yin Tang, EX-HN-3), GV-16 (Du Mai 16), and GV-20 (Du Mai 20).

Action in TCM: Supports the ear.

GB-14 Yang Bai

"Yang White"

Location: 1 Cun above the middle of the eyebrow, right above the pupil when looking straight ahead (▶ **Fig. 12.6**).

The total distance between mid-eyebrow and frontal hairline is 3 Cun; GB-14 is located at the end of the first third of this distance.

! Note

In case of baldness, the border of the original hairline can be demonstrated by frowning.

Depth of needling: 0.3 to 0.5 Cun, subcutaneously toward the pain site (site of function disorder).

Indication: Cephalgia, trigeminal neuralgia, sinusitis, vision disorders.

GB-14 is particularly sensitive to pressure with disorders in the gallbladder region (conspicuous trigger point).

The combination of GB-14 and GB-20 also with GB-8 improves the flow through the head in the sense of front–back coupling.

J. Bischko: Test point for gallbladder disorders.

Action in TCM: Supports the eyes.

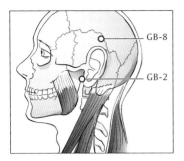

▶ **Fig. 12.5** GB-2 and GB-8.

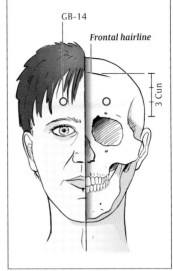

GB-14

Frontal hairline

3 Cun

▶ **Fig. 12.6** GB-14.

GB-20 Feng Chi

"Wind Pool"

Location: In a depression between the insertions of the sternocleidomastoid muscle and trapezius muscle at the lower edge of the occiput (▶ Fig. 12.7).

The needle is inserted at the level between occiput and atlas (upper head joints) in the region of the transverse process of the atlas; it passes through the splenius muscle of the head, then through the semispinalis muscle of the head, and becomes positioned close to the superior and inferior oblique muscles of the head.

Depth of needling: Approximately 1 Cun in the direction of the contralateral eye socket or the contralateral upper incisor region (depending on head position).

❗ Note
The vertebral artery is located at a considerable depth of 4 cm (often more). GB-20 is usually needled deeply, since this is often required to create a De Qi sensation. In slim patients, however, depth of needling should not exceed 2 cm.

Indication: All disorders with symptoms that resemble Wind: they appear suddenly and vary in localization and intensity (e.g., cervical syndrome, facial paresis, tinnitus, conjunctivitis, allergies, influenza or flulike infections).

J. Bischko: Master point for Wind disorders, Master point of the sympathetic nervous system, for all disorders where we find an overshooting reaction of the sympathetic nervous system (hypertension, tinnitus, vertigo, vegetative dysregulation, influenza or other infections, migraine), tension in the body (affecting the overall tone of the body) such as migraine, tension headache, premenstrual syndrome, dysmenorrhea, as well as vertigo and imbalance (regulation of balance).

This point is often needled in combination with BL-10, the Master Point of the parasympathetic nervous system (J. Bischko).

This point's localization explains the positive effect of GB-20 on tension in the neck muscles of the head joint region as well as blockage of the head joints. Via reflexes, afferent nerves from the head joint region effect:
- autonomic regulation (there are neural connections to autonomic centers)

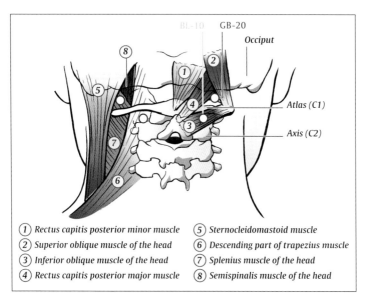

BL-10   GB-20
Occiput

Atlas (C1)

Axis (C2)

① Rectus capitis posterior minor muscle   ⑤ Sternocleidomastoid muscle
② Superior oblique muscle of the head   ⑥ Descending part of trapezius muscle
③ Inferior oblique muscle of the head   ⑦ Splenius muscle of the head
④ Rectus capitis posterior major muscle   ⑧ Semispinalis muscle of the head

▶ **Fig. 12.7** GB-20.

- overall tone of the body (by affecting the gamma system that controls overall body tone)
- regulation of balance (the upper cervical spine, in particular, is an important peripheral organ of balance)

Points in the head joint region can explain many of the indications listed above. They also provide a conventional medical explanation for J. Bischko's term "Master Point of the sympathetic nervous system" (BL-10).

Action in TCM:
- Eliminates Wind and Heat
- Slows ascending Liver Yang
- Clears the Mind (Shen) and opens the senses

GB-21 Jian Jing

"Shoulder Well"

Location: In the middle of the line connecting the acromion with the spinous process of C7, on the dorsal vertical extension of the mammillary line (▶ Fig. 12.8).

🔔 Note

How to localize C7: the first spinous process of the cervical spine that does not slide ventrally upon retroflexion of the head. During palpation, with the head in anteflexion, first search for the most prominent spinous process (probably C7) and mark it with the tip of the finger. If the finger remains in place while the head now moves into retroflexion, you have located C7; if, however, the finger moves in a ventral direction, you have located C6. Another possibility is to use two fingers for the examination: one finger is placed on the presumed C6 spinous process, the other on the C7 spinous process. Upon retroflexion, one can feel the ventral gliding of the upper spinous process and the two spinous processes approaching each other.

Depth of needling: 0.5 to 1 Cun, perpendicularly to the skin surface, or by using the dry-needling method.

┌─ Caution ─────────────
│ Deep needling can cause
│ pneumothorax in the first
│ intercostal space (ICS 1).
└────────────────────────

Indication: Shoulder and neck pain, headache, facilitation of childbirth, retained placenta, lactation disorders, mastitis.

GB-21 corresponds to a common trigger point.

Action in TCM:
- Removes obstructions in the channel
- Relaxes ligaments and tendons

GB-30 Huan Tiao

"Jumping Round" ("Circular Jump")

Location: Lateral side of the hip, on the connecting line between the greater trochanter and sacral hiatus, between the outer and middle third of the line (▶ Fig. 12.9). In China, this point is always needled with the patient in the lateral position. Hip and knee of the side to be treated are flexed, while the other leg beneath is extended.

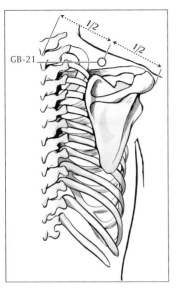

Depth of needling: 1.5 to 3 Cun, perpendicularly.

Indication: Lumbago, lumbago–sciatica syndrome; neuralgia-like symptoms and paresis of the lower extremity, coxalgia.

Action in TCM: Removes obstructions in the channel.

▶ **Fig. 12.8** GB-21.

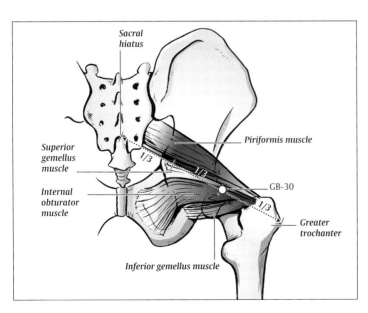

▶ **Fig. 12.9** GB-30.

GB-34 Yang Ling Quan

"Yang Mound Spring," Lower Sea Point (Lower He Point) of the Gallbladder, Master Point of the Muscles and Tendons

Location: In the depression in front of and below the head of the fibula (▶ **Fig. 12.10**).

🔒 **Note**

To find this point, first search for the head of the fibula in the region where the trouser seam would be. Then grip the head of the fibula between the index and middle fingers, with both fingers sliding caudally. GB-34 is located under the index finger, directly below and in front of the head of the fibula. Needling takes place in the direction of the interosseous membrane, that is, between the tibia and fibula. When the knee is flexed, the head of the fibula can be located by following the course of the clearly palpable tendon of the biceps muscle of the thigh, which runs toward the head of the fibula.

🔧 **Practical Tip**

Needling GB-34 may irritate deep fibers of the deep fibular nerve. Puncture of the common fibular nerve is also possible if it is located high up.

Depth of needling: 1 to 2 Cun, obliquely toward the interosseous membrane (between the tibia and fibula).

Indication: Myalgia, gonalgia, coxalgia, pain and paresis in the lower extremity, tinnitus, cephalgia, hypertension.

Action in TCM:
• Supports tendons and joints
• Regulates Liver Qi

GB-39 Xuan Zhong

"Suspended Bell", Channels of the Foot, Master Point of the Bone Marrow

Location: 3 Cun above the highest prominence of the lateral malleolus, at the anterior edge of the fibula (▶ **Fig. 12.11**). Chinese literature (Chinese Acupuncture and Moxibustion) sometimes localizes GB-39 at the posterior edge of the fibula. The decision is made by palpating for pressure sensitivity.

Depth of needling: 0.5 to 2 Cun, perpendicularly.

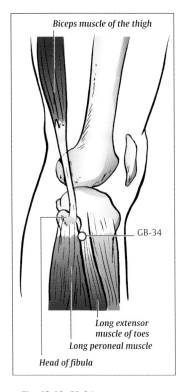

▶ **Fig. 12.10** GB-34.

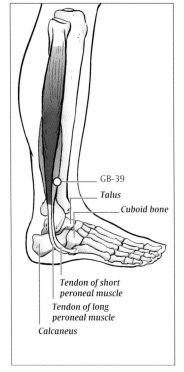

▶ **Fig. 12.11** GB-39.

Indication: Acute torticollis, cephalgia (Repletion), cervical syndrome.

🔳 Note
As a Group Luo Point of the three Yang channels of the foot, GB-39 affects disturbances of all three axes. This explains the particularly good effect on combined disturbances of anteflexion and retroflexion/lateroflexion as well

as rotation. These play a role, for example, in acute torticollis as well as in intercostal neuralgia.

Action in TCM:
- Supports Essence (Jing)
- Nourishes the marrow

GB-41 Zu Lin Qi

"Foot Overlooking Tears" ("Above Tears"), Opening Point of the Extraordinary Channel, Dai Mai (Girdle Vessel)

Location: At the body–base transition of the fourth and fifth metatarsal bones, lateral to the tendon of the long extensor muscle of toes running toward the little toe (▶ **Fig. 12.12**).

🛈 Note
The most accurate way to find the base of the fifth metatarsal bone is from the lateral edge of the foot. Starting at the clearly palpable base, palpate distal to the body–base transition of the fifth metatarsal bone. From here, continue in a medial direction along the extended line between the fourth and fifth toe. At this point, if indicated, GB-41 is clearly pressure sensitive.

Depth of needling: 0.3 to 0.5 Cun, perpendicularly.

Indication: Migraine, joint disorders, pain in the lateral regions of the head, thorax, and abdomen, mastitis, lumbago–sciatica syndrome.

Action in TCM:
- Regulates Liver Qi flow
- Eliminates Heat and Dampness

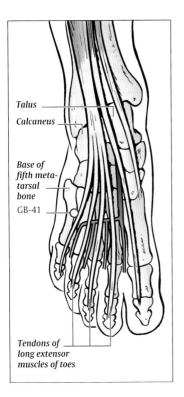

Talus
Calcaneus
Base of
fifth meta-
tarsal
bone
GB-41
Tendons of
long extensor
muscles of toes

▶ **Fig. 12.12** GB-41.

13 Liver Channel

▶ Fig. 13.1

Major Points

- LR-2: Sedation point
- LR-3: Source point (Yuan Point)
- LR-13: Front collecting point (Mu Point) of the spleen. Master point of the Zang organs
- LR-14: Front collecting point (Mu Point) of the liver

Associated Points

- LR-14: Front collecting point (Mu Point) of the liver
- BL-18: Back transport point (Back Shu Point) of the liver

Coupling Relationships

▶ Fig. 13.2

Top-to-bottom coupling: Pericardium–liver

Yin-Yang coupling: Liver–gallbladder

LR-2 Xing Jian

"Moving Between" ("Between Columns"), Sedation Point

Location: Proximal to the end of the interdigital fold between the first and second toes (▶ Fig. 13.3).

Depth of needling: 0.5 to 1 Cun, perpendicularly.

Indication: Spasmodic pain (especially in the gynecological area), cephalgia, glaucoma, pain and paresis in the lower extremity, thoracodynia, vertigo, tinnitus, sleep disorders.

Action in TCM:

- Cools Heat and drains Fire (with acute Repletion patterns)
- Cools Blood Heat

LR-3 Tai Chong

"Supreme Surge" ("Great Rush"), Source Point (Yuan Point)

Location: In the proximal corner between first and second metatarsal bones, where body and base regions of both bones approach each other (▶ Fig. 13.3).

Depth of needling: 0.5 to 1 Cun, perpendicularly, possibly in a slightly proximal direction.

Indication: Spasmolytic effect (often used in combination with

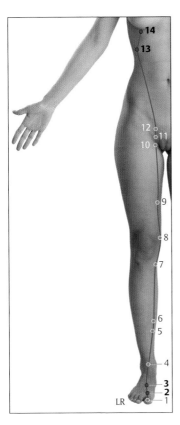

▶ **Fig. 13.1** Major points of the Liver Channel.

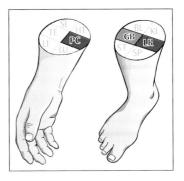

▶ **Fig. 13.2** Coupling relationships of the Liver Channel.

LR-2), cephalgia, obstipation, diarrhea, "liver and gallbladder problems," important distant point for the urogenital region, hypertension, vertigo, eye disorders.

Action in TCM:

* Regulates Liver Qi and Blood Stagnation
* Cools Heat in liver and gallbladder
* Calms Shen

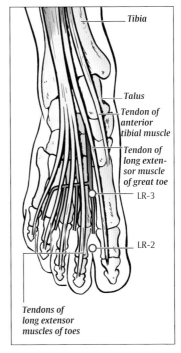

▶ **Fig. 13.3** LR-2 and LR-3.

LR-13 Zhang Men

"Camphorwood Gate" ("Bright Door"), Front Collecting Point (Mu Point) of the Spleen, Master Point of the Zang Organs

Location: At the free end of the 11th rib, at the lateral side of the abdomen (▶ **Fig. 13.4**).

Depth of needling: 0.5 Cun, obliquely.

Indication: Liver and gallbladder disorders, digestive disorders, metabolic disorders, vomiting.

Action in TCM: Tonifies Spleen.

LR-14 Qi Men

"Cycle Gate" ("Cycle Door"), Front Collecting Point (Mu Point) of the Liver

Location: In the sixth intercostal space (ICS 6) below the mammilla on the mammillary line (▶ **Fig. 13.4**).

🛈 Note
How to localize the ICS: Find the clearly palpable transition of sternal manubrium to sternal body. Lateral to it is the second rib, and below that is ICS 2.

Depth of needling: 0.5 Cun, obliquely along the course of the rib.

Indication: Liver disease, digestive disorders, intercostal neuralgia, vertigo.

Action in TCM: Regulates liver function.

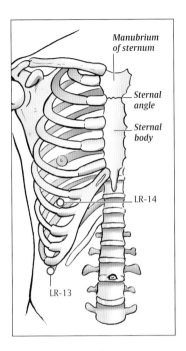

▶ **Fig. 13.4** LR-13 and LR-14.

14 Conception Vessel (Ren Mai)

▶ Fig. 14.1

Major Points

- CV-3: Front collecting point (Mu Point) of the bladder
- CV-4: Front collecting point (Mu Point) of the small intestine
- CV-6: General tonification point
- CV-8: General tonification point
- CV-12: Front collecting point (Mu Point) of the stomach. Master point of the Fu organs. Front collecting point (Mu Point) of the Middle Energizer
- CV-17: Front collecting point (Mu Point) of the pericardium. Master point of the respiratory tract. Front collecting point (Mu Point) of the Upper Energizer
- CV-22: Local point
- CV-24: Local point

Associated Points

- LU-7: Opening point of the Conception Vessel

CV-3 Zhong Ji

"Central Pole" ("Middle Extreme"), Front Collecting Point (Mu Point) of the Bladder

Location: 1 Cun cranial to the middle of the upper edge of the symphysis (▶ **Fig. 14.2**).

🛈 Note
When using Cun as a measure in the abdominal region, it is very important to take the total distance between the upper edge of the symphysis and the navel—5 Cun—as guidance. This is the only way of taking into account the differences in abdominal girth, which cannot be accomplished using the usual thumb–Cun measure.

Depth of needling: 1 to 1.5 Cun, perpendicularly.

Indication: Urogenital tract disorders, incontinence, menstruation disorders (such as dysmenorrhea, amenorrhea, irregular menstruation), female infertility, vaginal discharge, postpartum hemorrhage, postpartum

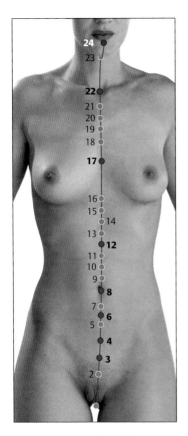

► **Fig. 14.1** Major points of the Conception Vessel.

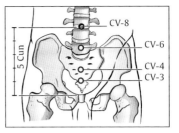

► **Fig. 14.2** CV-3.

afterpains, pain and itching of the exterior genitals, erectile dysfunction, premature ejaculation.

Action in TCM: Regulates and nourishes kidney and bladder.

CV-4 Guan Yuan

"Pass Head" ("Energy Pass"),
Front Collecting Point (Mu Point)
of the Small Intestine

Location: 2 Cun cranial to the middle of the upper edge of the symphysis (for precise orientation, see CV-3 (p.116) (▶ **Fig. 14.3**)).

🔋 Note
CV-4 represents the intersection of the interior branches of the Three Yin Channels of the Foot. This explains the broad effect on gynecological and urogenital tract disorders, similar to the effect of SP-6 (intersection of the exterior, point-carrying parts of the Three Yin Channels of the Foot).

Depth of needling: 1 to 1.5 Cun, perpendicularly.

Indication: Pre-eminent point for treating urogenital and gyneco-logical disorders; important toni-fication point for emotional, mental and physical exhaustion, abdominal complaints, persistent postpartum hemorrhage.
   König/Wancura: CV-4 + SP-6: basic point combination for uro-genital tract disorders.

Action in TCM:
- Tonifies and nourishes:
  – Kidneys and Original Qi (Yuan Qi)
  – Blood, Yin, and Essence (Jing)

CV-6 Qi Hai

"Sea of Qi" ("Energy Sea")

Location: 1.5 Cun below the navel (for precise orientation, see CV-3 (p.116) (▶ **Fig. 14.3**)).

Depth of needling: 1 to 1.5 Cun, perpendicularly.

Indication: Pre-eminent tonifica-tion point for emotional, mental and physical exhaustion, often used with moxa; exhaustion, cir-culatory dysregulation, erectile dysfunction.

Action in TCM:
- Tonifies and nourishes: Qi and Yang (especially with moxa)
- Regulates Qi and harmonizes Blood Flow

CV-8 Shen Que

"Spirit Gate Tower" ("Navel")

Location: In the center of the navel (▶ **Fig. 14.4**).

🔋 Note
One possibility of providing energy in case of general states of exhaustion is to apply navel moxibustion with ginger and salt (three Yang substances).

Indication: Absolutely no nee-dling! Moxibustion is frequently useful for general tonification.

Action in TCM: Tonifies and nourishes Qi and Yang (using moxibustion).

CV-12 Zhong Wan

"Central Stomach Duct" ("Center of Power"), Front Collecting Point (Mu Point) of the Stomach, Master Point of the Fu Organs, Front Collecting Point (Mu Point) of the Middle Energizer

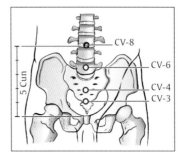

▶ **Fig. 14.3** CV-4 and CV-6.

Location: At the midpoint of a line connecting the base of the xiphoid with the navel (▶ **Fig. 14.4**).

🔲 Note
As with the lower abdomen, it is important for points in the upper abdomen to take the distance between the base of the xiphoid (intersection of costal arches) and the navel—8 Cun—as guidance for points. This is the only way to take into account the differences in abdominal girth.

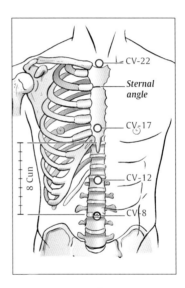

▶ **Fig. 14.4** CV-8 and CV-12.

Depth of needling: 1 to 1.5 Cun, perpendicularly.

Indication: Pre-eminent point for all gastrointestinal tract disorders; gastritis, ulcers of stomach and duodenum, meteorism, Roemheld syndrome (gastrocardiac syndrome), nausea, vomiting, singultus (hiccup), sleep disorders.

Action in TCM:
- Tonifies and nourishes: Stomach Qi and Spleen Qi
- Removes Stomach Qi Stagnation

CV-17 Shan Zhong

"Chest Center" ("Sea of Tranquility"), Front Collecting Point (Mu Point) of the Pericardium, Master Point of the Respiratory Tract, Front Collecting Point (Mu Point) of the Upper Energizer

Location: On the median line at the level of the mammilla, in ICS 4 (▶ Fig. 14.5).

❗ Note

The distance between the upper edge of the sternal manubrium and the base of the xiphoid measures 9 Cun. However, orientation in the area of the ventral thorax usually takes place by determining the intercostal space.

Depth of needling: 0.3 to 0.5 Cun, subcutaneously in a caudal direction toward the tip of the xiphoid process, or in a lateral direction toward the mammilla.

❗ Note

Anatomically, the osseous lamina in the region of CV-17 may be very thin (due to disturbed sternal ossification during embryonic development). There may even be foramina present. This creates the risk of intracardiac puncture. A more or less highly developed sternal foramen is found in 8 to 10% of the population. Thin osseous lamina or connective-tissue membrane may render the results of the palpation inconspicuous. The distance between the skin surface and the dorsal surface of the sternum measures only 12 to 22 mm. Cases of death have been reported. Therefore, needling should be strictly tangential. For palpation of ICS 4, it is recommended to search first for the clearly palpable transition of the sternal angle between sternal manubrium and sternal corpus. Lateral to it is the second rib, caudal to it is ICS 2.

Indication: Pre-eminent point for acute and chronic breathing disorders, bronchial asthma, bronchitis, dyspnea, thoracodynia, functional heart problems, sensation of tightness in the thorax.

Action in TCM:
- Regulates Qi and opens the thorax
- Descends rebellious Lung Qi and Stomach Qi
- Strengthens Qi, especially the thorax breath Qi

CV-22 Tian Tu

"Celestial Chimney" ("Sky Prominence")

Location: In the middle of the jugular notch of the sternum, at the level of the attachment of the clavicle (▶ Fig. 14.5).

Method of needling: According to Chinese literature, for acute asthma attacks, CV-22 is needled deeply retrosternally.

Depth of needling: 0.5 to 1 Cun, retrosternally.

Indication: Bronchial asthma, singultus (hiccup), globus sensation, hoarseness.

— Caution —
In case of needling too deeply and in patients with infections, there is a risk of mediastinitis because of interconnecting spaces in the connective tissue.

Action in TCM:
- Strengthens the voice
- Descends rebellious Lung Qi

CV-24 Cheng Jiang

"Sauce Receptacle" ("Receiving Saliva")

Location: Deepest site of the mandibular median line, in the middle of the mentolabial crease (▶ Fig. 14.6).

🔒 Note
If needling is carried out for the purpose of reducing the pharyngeal reflex (e.g., during endoscopic examination or taking of dental casts), it is recommended to use a very short needle prior to the examination. If the needle is bent at a right angle in the area of the handle, it can remain in place during examination.

Depth of needling: 0.2 to 0.3 Cun, perpendicularly.

Indication: Facial pain, toothache, facial paresis, trigeminal neuralgia, hypersalivation, facial spasm,

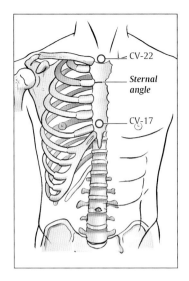

▶ **Fig. 14.5** CV-17 and CV-22.

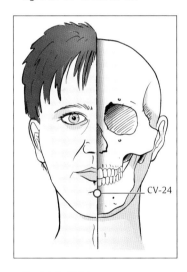

▶ **Fig. 14.6** CV-24.

reduction of pharyngeal reflex for endoscopic examination as well as dental procedures (taking a cast).

Action in TCM: Eliminates exterior and interior Wind.

15 Governing Vessel (Du Mai)

Major Points

▶ Fig. 15.1, ▶ Fig. 15.2

- GV-4: General tonification point
- GV-14: Convergence of all Yang Channels
- GV-15: Local point
- GV-16: Local point
- GV-20: Local point with systemic effect
- GV-26: Local point, emergency point

Associated Points

SI-3: Opening point of the Governing Vessel.

GV-4 Ming Men

"Life Gate"

Location: Below the spinous process of L2 (▶ Fig. 15.3).

GV-4 is located at the same level as BL-23. An interior branch of the Kidney Channel joins here. GV-4 therefore enhances the effect of BL-23.

ℹ **Additional Information**
The literature describes very rare cases of injuries to the spinal cord following extremely deep needling in a cranial direction. If the needle is inserted in the described direction, insertion depth should therefore not exceed 1 Cun, and the needle should be guided perpendicularly or in a slightly caudal direction.

❗ Note
GV-4 as well as BL-23 have a tonifying effect on dysfunctions of the kidney and bladder. They are indicated in patients with symptoms of Cold, Weakness, and Vacuity. For concurrent lumbago, needling or moxibustion of this "dorsal tonification line for lumbago" is recommended. If appropriate (when sensitive to pressure), additional needling or moxibustion of BL-52 (1.5 Cun lateral to BL-23) is an option. Instead of needling BL-23 and BL-52 as described, moxa pads or other self-heating, scent-neutral plasters may also be used.

Depth of needling: 0.5 to 1 Cun, perpendicularly or, possibly, in an oblique caudal direction.

Indication: Pre-eminent point for tonifying Yang and especially Kidney Yang; lumbago, urogenital disorders, sexual dysfunction, tinnitus, cephalgia.

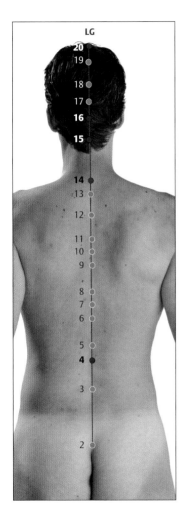

▶ **Fig. 15.1** Major channels of the Governing Vessel (1).

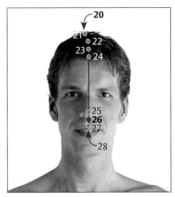

▶ **Fig. 15.2** Major channels of the Governing Vessel (2).

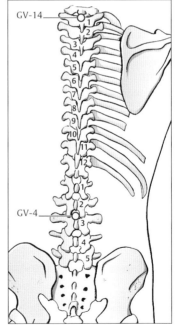

▶ **Fig. 15.3** GV-4.

Action in TCM:

- Tonifies and nourishes:
  - Kidney functional circle and Original Qi (Yuan Qi)
  - Blood, Yin, and Essence (Jing)

GV-14 Da Zhui

"Great Hammer"

Location: Below the spinous process of C7 (► Fig. 15.4).

🔔 Note

How to locate the spinous process of C7: Unlike C6, C7 does not slide ventrally when reclining the head. Examine by placing the middle and index fingers on the supposed spinous processes of C6 and C7. If the fingers are positioned correctly, they move toward each other when the head is reclined, and the upper spinous process swerves in a ventral direction.

Depth of needling: 0.5 to 1 Cun, perpendicularly.

Indication: Cephalgia; immune modulation; fever, paralysis, tinnitus.

J. Bischko: Convergence ("reunion") point with connections to the six Fu organs. (In combination with other points, this point is also called the "spider.")

GV-14 affects all Yang channels. Quick orientation in case of headache and neck pain can be obtained by palpating the major points of the "spider" around GV-14.

🔔 Note

Not all points of the "spider" are needled simultaneously. Select only the points that are most sensitive to pressure.

Action in TCM:
- Clears Heat
- Tonifies and nourishes: Yang and Defense Qi (Wei Qi)

GV-15 Ya Men

"Mute's Gate" ("Dumb Gate")

Location: Above the spinous process of C2, at the same level as BL-10, 0.5 Cun above the dorsal hairline (► Fig. 15.5).

🔔 Note

When needling both GV-15 and GV-16: Needle in a slightly caudal direction while the patient's head is bent slightly forward. The tip of the needle should be positioned in the nuchal ligament. Do not stimulate. If GV-16 is needled too deeply, there is a risk of penetrating into the cerebellomedullary cistern.

Depth of needling: 0.5 Cun, in a slightly caudal direction.

Indication: Important point for speech disorders, especially in children; aphasia, general speech disorders, epilepsy, apoplexy, cervical syndrome, stiffness of the neck, occipital pain.

Action in TCM: Strengthens the senses and the Mind (Shen).

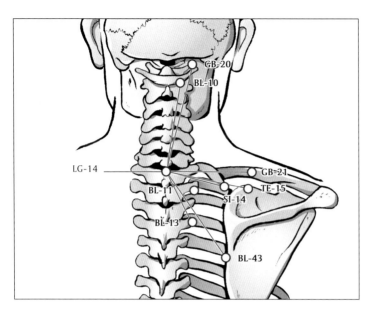

▶ **Fig. 15.4** GV-14.

GV-16 Feng Fu

"Wind Mansion" ("Windy Mansion")

Location: Below the exterior occipital protuberance, at the same level as GB-20 (▶ **Fig. 15.5**).

🔒 **Note**
See GV-15 (p. 124).

Depth of needling: 0.5 Cun, in a slightly caudal direction (see GV-15 (p. 124)).

Indication: Cephalgia; promotes longitudinal flow through the head (in combination with EX-HN-1); tinnitus, confusion; pre-

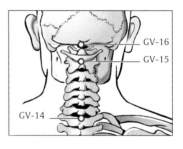

▶ **Fig. 15.5** GV-15 and GV-16.

eminent point for exterior and interior Wind disorders; vertigo, rhinitis, sinusitis.

Action in TCM: Expels exterior and interior Wind.

GV-20 Bai Hui

"Hundred Convergences"

Location: On the median line of the head, 5 Cun into the scalp from the frontal hair line, on a line connecting the tips of both ears. In German-language literature, the ear axis (▶ **Fig. 15.6**) is often pointed out as a guide for localizing the tip of the ear and the connecting line.

Depth of needling: 0.5 Cun, subcutaneously toward the front or the back.

Indication: Important sedation point; mental and emotional harmonization; cephalgia, sleep disorders, vertigo, symptoms of anxiety (apart from LI-4 and ST-36, one of the most often used points).

Action in TCM:
- Calms interior Wind
- Harmonizes and sedates and/or calms the Mind (Shen)

GV-26 Shui Gou

"Water Trough," also known as "Ren Zhong," "Middle of Person" ("Middle of Man")

Location: In the philtrum on the anterior median line, at the transition from the nasal third and the remaining two-thirds of the connecting line between nose and upper lip margin (▶ **Fig. 15.7**).

Depth of needling: 0.5 Cun, obliquely in a cranial direction.

Indication: Collapse, epileptic seizure, acute lumbago.

⚠ Note

With the above indications, in emergency situations (when no needles are available), apply acupressure by pressing the thumb firmly against the lower edge of the nose.

Action in TCM: Strengthens the senses.

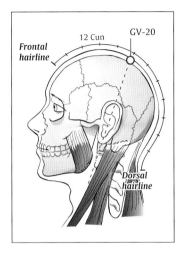

▶ **Fig. 15.6** GV-20.

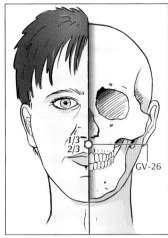

▶ **Fig. 15.7** GV-26.

16 Extra Points

In China there has been an official agreement since 1991, in coordination with the World Health Organization (WHO), on 48 Extra Points. These Extra Points are named after the respective region of the body (▶ Table 16.1, ▶ Table 16.2), and their number varies from region to region.

▶ Table 16.1

English names	Number of points
EX-HN (**H**ead–**N**eck)	15
EX-CA (**C**hest–**A**bdomen)	1
EX-B (**B**ack)	9
EX-UE (**U**pper **E**xtremity)	11
EX-LE (**L**ower **E**xtremity)	12

► Table 16.2

Chinese name	English name	Chinese Acupuncture and Moxibustion
Shi Shen Cong	EX-HN-1	Extra 6
Yin Tang	EX-HN-3	Extra 2
Yu Yao	EX-HN-4	Extra 5
Tai Yang	EX-HN-5	Extra 1
Jing Bai Lao	EX-HN-15	Extra 16
Ding Chuan	EX-B-1	Extra 14
Hua Tuo Jia Ji	EX-B-2	Extra 15
Shi Qi Zhui	EX-B-8	Extra 18
Wai Lao Gong/Luo Zhen	EX-UE-8	Extra 28
Ba Xie	EX-UE-9	Extra 27
He Ding	EX-LE-2	Extra 38
Nei Xi Yan	EX-LE-4	-
Xi Yan	EX-LE-5	Extra 37
Lan Wei Xue	EX-LE-7	Extra 39
Ba Feng	EX-LE-10	Extra 40

EX-HN-1 Si Shen Cong

"Alert Spirit Quartet"

Location: Si Shen Cong consists of four points, which lie 1 Cun frontal, dorsal, and lateral, respectively, to GV-20 (▸ **Fig. 16.1**).

Depth of needling: Each point is needled 0.5 to 1 Cun subcutaneously outward (not inward).

Indication: Restlessness, nervousness (sedative effect, similar to GV-20), vertigo, headache, sleep disorders; increases effect of GV-20.

Combinations: Sleep disorders: EX-HN-1 + HT-7 + SP-6.
Nausea, vomiting: EX-HN-1 + PC-6 + ST-36.

Action in TCM: Calms the Mind (Shen).

EX-HN-3 Yin Tang

"Hall of Impression"

Location: In the middle between the eyebrows (▸ **Fig. 16.2**).
J. Bischko localizes this point deeper at the root of the nose.

Depth of needling: Approximately 1 Cun, subcutaneously in a caudal direction toward the root of the nose.

> 🔲 **Practical Tip**
> To needle EX-HN-3, lift up a skin fold between the eyebrows and move the needle subcutaneously in a caudal direction toward the root of the nose. Forming a skin fold over the glabella allows the needle to be pushed forward without discomfort.

Indication: Headache, especially frontal and tension headache, eye disorders, rhinitis, sinusitis, sleep disorders.
In French nomenclature, Yin Tang is called PdM (Point de Merveille). This refers to the quick action this point has on rhinitis and headache.

Combinations: According to J. Bischko, the Yin Tang (EX-HN-3) and BL-2 form the "ventral magic triangle." The ventral magic triangle has a relaxing effect, especially in case of headache, rhinitis, and sinusitis. The two BL-2 points are needled perpendicularly, or with the tip of the needle directed toward the root of the nose (in the same direction as EX-HN-3).

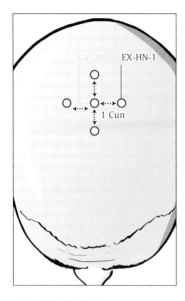

▶ **Fig. 16.1** EX-HN-1.

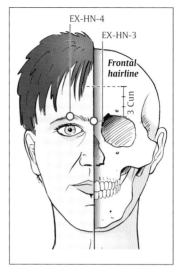

▶ **Fig. 16.2** EX-HN-3 and EX-HN-4.

Action in TCM:

- Relieves the nose
- Eliminates Wind

EX-HN-4 Yu Yao

"Fish's Lumbus"

Location: In the middle of the eyebrow, above the pupil when looking straight ahead (▶ **Fig. 16.2**).

Depth of needling: 0.5 Cun, sub-cutaneously toward the medial or lateral end of the eyebrow.

Indication: Eye disorders, frontal headache, facial paresis, trigeminal neuralgia.

Action in TCM: Improves vision.

EX-HN-5 Tai Yang

"Greater Yang"

Location: In a depression approximately 1 Cun posterior (towards the ear) from the middle of the connecting line between the outer end of the eyebrow and the lateral corner of the eye (▶ **Fig. 16.3**).

Depth of needling: Approx. 0.5 Cun, perpendicularly or subcutaneously toward the temple.

🔒 Note
There is usually a distinct palpable depression. Patients like to press this point themselves in case of headache. If pressure is a pleasant sensation, Tai Yang can be used to treat even acute headaches locally. (Otherwise use distant points for acute headaches.)

Indication: Headache, especially migraine, eye disorders, trigeminal neuralgia, facial paresis.

Action in TCM:
- Relieves pain
- Improves vision

EX-HN-15 Jing Bai Lao

"Hundred Taxations"

Location: 2 Cun cranial to the tip of the spinous process of C7 and 1 Cun lateral to the median line (▶ **Fig. 16.4**).

🔒 Note
The distance between the dorsal hairline and the lower edge of the spinous process of C7 measures 3 Cun.

Depth of needling: 0.5 to 1 Cun, in a slightly caudal direction.

Indication: Cervical syndrome, spastic torticollis, fixed torticollis.

Action in TCM: Harmonizes the flow of Qi.

EX-B-1 Ding Chuan

"Gasping"

Location: 0.5 Cun lateral to GV-14 (lateral to the tip of the spinous process of C7; ▶ **Fig. 16.5**).

Depth of needling: 0.5 to 1 Cun, in the direction of the spinal column, or sagittal in a slightly caudal direction.

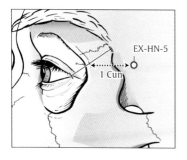

▶ **Fig. 16.3** EX-HN-5.

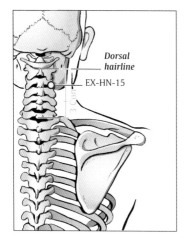

▶ **Fig. 16.4** EX-HN-15.

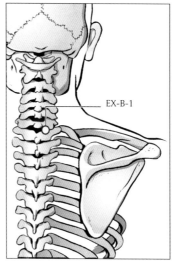

▶ **Fig. 16.5** EX-B-1.

Indication: Disorders of the respiratory tract.

Action in TCM: Regulates lung function.

EX-B-2 Hua Tuo Jia Ji

"Hua Tuo's Paravertebral Points"
According to Hua Tuo

Location: A series of 17 points on each side of the spinal column, 0.5 Cun lateral to the tip of the spinous processes of T1 to L5 (▶ Fig. 16.6). These points, therefore, are located at the same level as the points of the interior branch of the Bladder Channel.

🔳 Note

The Hua Tuo Points lie in the region of the small vertebral joints (facet joints). This explains their effect on dysfunctions in that region. With dysfunctions in the cervical area, pressure-sensitive sites can be found along the line of Hua Tao Points also in a cervical direction. These sites represent myogelosis in the area of the paravertebral back muscles that developed as a result of segmental dysfunctions and should be treated.

Depth of needling: 0.3 to 0.5 Cun, obliquely against the vertebrae.

🔳 Note

When needling the points of the interior branch of the Bladder Channel at an angle of 45° in a median direction, the needle tips reach the area of the Hua Tuo Points (enhancing the effect).

Indication: Local pain in the region of the spinal column, chronic dysfunction of internal organs.

Action in TCM: Relieves pain and dysfunction.

EX-B-8 Shi Qi Zhui

"Seventeenth Vertebra Point" (counted from T1)

Location: Below the tip of the spinous process of L5 (▶ Fig. 16.7).

🔳 Note

Shi Qi Zhui is located in the region of the lumbar–sacral transition, where instabilities, in particular, play a major role. Instability represents a contraindication for manipulation (therapeutic approach of chiropractic). Acupuncture, however, offers the possibility of treating dysfunctions involving increased joint mobility (instability) and diminished joint mobility (blockage).

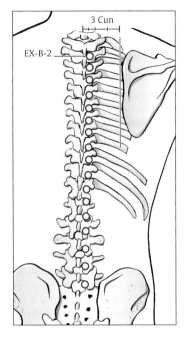

▸ **Fig. 16.6** EX-B-2.

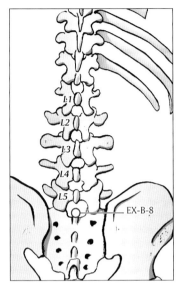

▸ **Fig. 16.7** EX-B-8.

Depth of needling: Approximately 0.5 Cun, slightly obliquely in a cranial direction into the area of the interspinal ligament (for details on depth of needling, see GV-4 (p. 122)).

Indication: Lumbago, lumbago–sciatica syndrome, menstruation disorders, vaginal hemorrhage; pelvic presentation (breech) during pregnancy, in combination with BL-67 (moxa).

🛇 Note
Do not perform (downward) descending stimulation during pregnancy.

Action in TCM: Relieves pain and dysfunction.

EX-UE-8 Wai Lao Gong

"External Crick in the Neck Point," also known as **"Luo Zhen," "Outer Laogong"**

Location: On the back of the hand, at the transition between the body and head of the second and third metacarpal bones, about 0.5 Cun proximal to the second and third metacarpophalangeal joints (▶ **Fig. 16.8**).

Depth of needling: 0.5 to 1 Cun, obliquely in a proximal direction, or perpendicularly.

Indication: Cervical syndrome, neck pain, shoulder pain.

Additional Information
König and Wancura describe PaM 108 = Luo Zhen in the same location as EX-UE-8 (Wai Lao Gong). PaM 108 is an important distant point for acute cervical syndrome and/or shoulder pain.

Action in TCM: Relieves pain and dysfunction.

EX-UE-9 Ba Xie

"Eight Evils"

Location: Four points on the back of each hand (▶ **Fig. 16.9**).

With the fist loosely clenched, these points are located proximal to the end of the folds between the fingers, at the border between the side of the hand and the palm.

Note
The best method for localizing the metacarpophalangeal joints is mild traction of the respective finger. This gently pulls in the skin in the joint area.

Depth of needling: 0.3 Cun, in a proximal direction, with fist loosely clenched.

Indication: Disorders of the metacarpophalangeal joints, headache, toothache, restlessness, osteoarthritis and arthritis in the fingers.

Action in TCM: Strengthens Wei Qi.

EX-LE-2 He Ding

"Crane Top"

Location: In the middle of the upper edge of the patella (▶ **Fig. 16.10**).

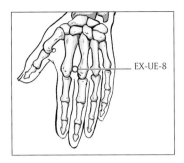

▶ **Fig. 16.8** EX-UE-8.

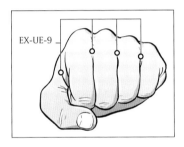

▶ **Fig. 16.9** EX-UE-9.

Depth of needling: Approximately 0.3 Cun, perpendicularly.

🔧 **Practical Tip**

When needling very deeply, there is a risk of puncturing the suprapatellar bursa and causing infections.

Indication: Pain and dysfunction in the knee area (wobbly knee, involuntary buckling of the knee).

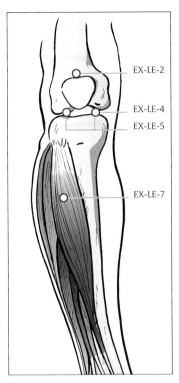

▶ **Fig. 16.10** EX-LE-2.

Combinations: Gonalgia: EX-LE-2 + ST-36 + GB-34 + SP-9.

Action in TCM: Relieves pain and dysfunction.

EX-LE-4 Nei Xi Yan

"Inner Eye of the Knee" (EX-LE-4 is part of EX-LE-5)

Location: When the knee is slightly bent, in the depression medial to the patellar ligament in the region of the inner "Eye of the Knee" (▶ **Fig. 16.11**).

Depth of needling: 0.3 Cun, perpendicularly, or approximately 0.5 Cun subcutaneously in the direction of ST-35 (see EX-LE-5 below).

Indication: Gonalgia.

Action in TCM: Relieves pain and dysfunction.

EX-LE-5 Xi Yan

"Eye of the Knee"

Location: Two points below the patella, medial and lateral to the patellar tendon: ST-35 and EX-LE-4. Therefore, EX-LE-4 is included in EX-LE-5 (▶ **Fig. 16.11**).

🚺 Note

These two points correspond to the puncture sites for arthroscopy. When needling deeply,

the needle tip may end up in an intra-articular position (Caution: Undesirable).

Depth of needling: Approximately 0.3 Cun, perpendicularly (see also EX-LE-4 above).

Indication: Pain and dysfunction (EX-LE-2) (p. 136)).

Combinations: Gonalgia: EX-LE-5 + EX-LE-2 + ST-36 + GB-34 + SP-9.

Action in TCM: Relieves pain and dysfunction.

EX-LE-7 Lan Wei Xue

"Appendix Point"

Location: On the Stomach Channel, 2 Cun distal to ST-36 (▶ **Fig. 16.11**).

Depth of needling: 1 to 1.5 Cun, perpendicularly.

Indication: Test point for appendicitis (important for diagnosis), pain and dysfunction in the leg area.

Action in TCM: Relieves pain and dysfunction.

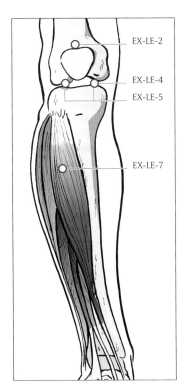

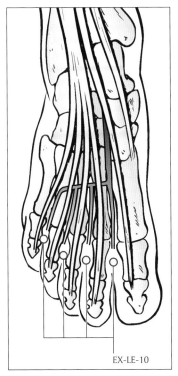

▶ **Fig. 16.11** EX-LE-4, EX-LE-5, and EX-LE-7.

▶ **Fig. 16.12** EX- LE-10.

EX-LE-10 Ba Feng

"Eight Winds"

Location: Four points on the back of the foot, proximal to the end of the interdigital creases, at the border between the side of the foot and the sole (▶ Fig. 16.12).

🔲 Note
The best way to localize the metacarpophalangeal joints is by mild traction of the respective toe. This pulls the skin in the joint area slightly inward.

Depth of needling: Approximately 3 Cun, in a slightly proximal direction.

Indication: Pain in the back of the foot.

Action in TCM:
- Expels Wind
- Relieves pain and dysfunction

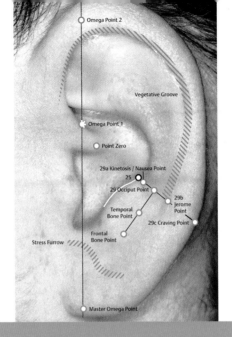

Part 2
Ear Acupuncture
Points

17 Anatomy of the Outer Ear (Auricula)

The helical brim (helix) forms the outer shape of the auricula (▶ Fig. 17.1). The helix originates at the bottom of the cavity of the concha and ascends as the root of the helix (crus of helix). Then follows the body of the helix which descends as the tail of the helix toward the ear lobe. The helix then turns into the ear lobe (auricular lobule). In the upper part of the helix, we usually find a protrusion or widening of the helical brim, namely the Darwinian tubercle (auricular hillock). Parallel to the helix runs the anthelix. It originates in the cranial part of the auricula with two limbs (crura of anthelix): the inferior anthelical crus and the superior anthelical crus. Between the two anthelical crura lies the triangular fossa. The anthelix turns into the antitragus in the lower part of the ear. The border between them is formed by the postantitragal fossa.

The scapha lies between the helix and the superior anthelical crus plus anthelix.

The tragus is bordered by the intertragic notch and the supratragic notch.

The cavity of the concha is located at the bottom of the auricula and is divided by the crus of helix into two parts: the superior concha (cymba) and the inferior concha.

The outer auditory canal (external acoustic meatus) is located in the inferior concha and is hidden from view by the tragus.

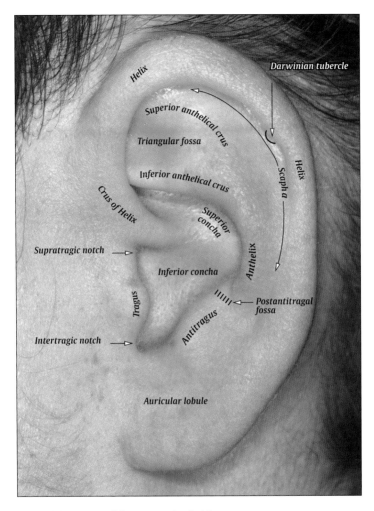

▶ **Fig. 17.1** Anatomy of the outer ear (auricula).

18 Zones of Auricular Innervation According to Nogier

The auricula (▶ **Fig. 18.1**) is innervated by three nerves:
- The auricular branch of the vagus nerve
- The auriculotemporal nerve of the trigeminal nerve
- The great auricular nerve of the cervical plexus

The auricular branch of the vagus nerve innervates the concha. The "endodermal organs" are projected here. The great auricular nerve of the cervical plexus supplies the lobule, the outer helical brim about as far as the Darwinian tubercle, and the back of the ear. These areas correspond to the ectodermal germ layer.

The remaining, and by far the largest, part of the ear is innervated by the auriculotemporal nerve of the trigeminal nerve. The "mesodermal organs" are projected here (▶ **Fig. 18.2**).

According to Nogier, the different zones are assigned to different functional areas:
- Endodermal zone → metabolism
- Mesodermal zone → motor function
- Ectodermal zone → head and central nervous system

In line with this tripartition, Nogier found control points for each functional area; these are the Omega Points.

 Auriculotemporal nerve of trigeminal nerve

 Auricular branch of vagus nerve

 Great auricular nerve of cervical plexus

▶ **Fig. 18.2** Auricular regulation points.

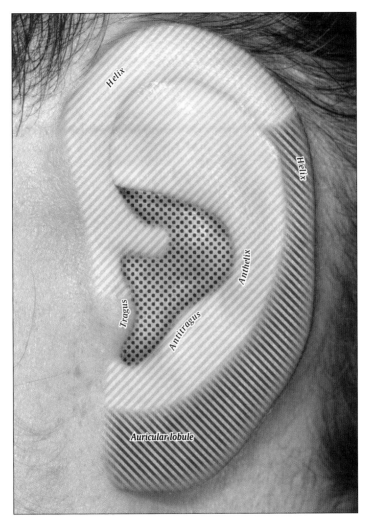

▶ **Fig. 18.1** Zones of auricular innervation according to Nogier.

19 Newer Research on Auricular Innervation

Newer research on ear innervation[95] documents a high density and number of nerve fibers in the outer ear compared to other regions of the head (▶ Fig. 19.1, ▶ Fig. 19.2). The auricula is supplied by four different nerves of branchiogenic as well as somatogenic origin:

- Great auricular nerve (cervical plexus)
- Auriculotemporal nerve (trigeminal nerve)
- Auricular branch of vagus nerve
- Lesser occipital nerve (cervical plexus)

Innervation by the great auricular nerve (cervical plexus) dominates the lateral surface of the outer ear. The anthelix is predominantly innervated either by the auricular branch of the vagus nerve only, partly by the great auricular nerve, or by both. The superior and inferior anthelical crura are predominantly supplied by the great auricular nerve. The lobule and the antitragus are primarily innervated by the great auricular nerve. The tragus is primarily supplied jointly by the great auricular nerve and the auriculotemporal nerve. The helix tail and scapha are almost always innervated by the great auricular nerve only. The helix spine is 90% innervated by the auriculotemporal nerve.

The superior concha (cymba) is consistently innervated by the auricular branch of the vagus nerve, while the inferior concha is innervated by that nerve in about half of all cases, while in the other half it is innervated by both the auricular branch of the vagus nerve and the greater auricular nerve. There are no areas of overlap between the innervation zones of the three nerves.

On the dorsal side, the lesser occipital nerve (▶ Fig. 19.4) participates in the innervation of the upper third of the ear, often jointly with the great auricular nerve.

The middle third is most frequently innervated by the great auricular nerve (▶ Fig. 19.3) and the auricular branch of the vagus

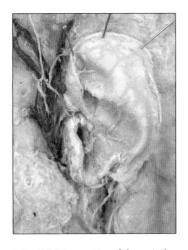

▶ **Fig. 19.1** Innervation of the auricula, side.

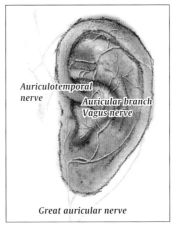

Auriculotemporal nerve

Auricular branch Vagus nerve

Great auricular nerve

▶ **Fig. 19.3** Great auricular nerve.

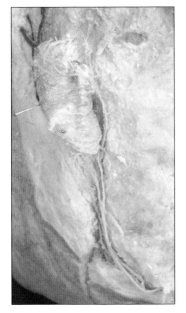

▶ **Fig. 19.2** Innervation of the auricula, back.

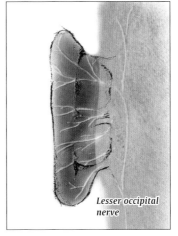

Lesser occipital nerve

▶ **Fig. 19.4** Lesser occipital nerve.

nerve. Less frequently, the lesser occipital nerve participates in the innervation. The lower third is almost always innervated by the great auricular nerve, less frequently by the auricular branch of the vagus nerve. The dorsal side also does not have any areas that are innervated by all three nerves.

Likewise, projections of the same organ are ascribed to different localization sites. For example, we find (a) projection zones that correspond to the organ parenchyma, (b) projection zones of the corresponding nerve innervation, and (c) projection zones representing the functional state of the organ.

Due to variations in auricular shape, it is conceivable that overlaps of innervation zones also vary individually. This means that the frequently described points are actually zones rather than points. The active ear acupuncture point needs to be searched for within those zones depending on individual circumstances. Credit for this approach certainly goes to Nogier, who tried to identify individual representations of acupuncture points through his auriculocardiac reflex model (ACR).

Nogier's Reflex (ACR, Auriculocardiac Reflex)

Underlying Nogier's reflex is a cutaneo-vascular reflex, which Nogier discovered in 1968. He noticed a change in the pulse wave of the radial artery when stimulating irritated ear points or zones. While doing so, he observed two phenomena: an increase in pulse strength, which he called positive ACR; and a decrease in pulse strength, which he called negative ACR. A positive ACR indicates an irritated (interference) zone in need of treatment.

For the school of Nogier, this is the most important approach when selecting acupuncture points. In this respect, the school of auricular medicine differs significantly from the Chinese school.

20 Topography of Reflex Zones

The distribution of ear acupuncture points on the auricula follows a certain pattern. Localization of individual organs or body regions corresponds to that in an inverted fetus (▶ Fig. 20.1, ▶ Fig. 20.2):

- The points in the area of the ear lobe connect with the head and face.
- The upper extremity projects in the area of the scapha.
- The points on the anthelix and anthelical crura connect with the trunk of the body and the lower extremity.
- The internal organs project in the cavity of the concha.
- According to Nogier, the lower extremity projects in the triangular fossa, whereas according to the Chinese school the pelvic organs project there.
- According to Nogier, the sympathetic innervation of the intestines projects on the crus of helix, while the Chinese school assigns this area to the diaphragm.

- The points related to hormonal activity are also assigned differently. The Chinese school describes only an endocrine region, while Nogier differentiates between hypothalamic projections of the adrenal, thyroid, parathyroid, and mammary glands.

These somewhat different anatomical settings are not necessarily contradictory. They may be understood as different reaction types and may be classified as functional or organo-pathological disorders. Nogier's points may often be assigned to organ-specific pathologies, while the Chinese school more likely describes functional relationships.

According to Nogier, the motor elements project on the back of the auricula and the sensory elements on the front of the auricula. This means that the motor zone of an organ on the back of the ear is located exactly opposite the sensory zone of that organ on the front of the ear.

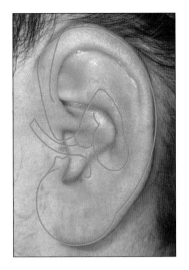

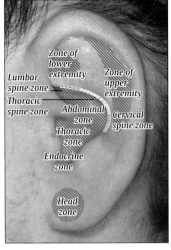

▶ **Fig. 20.1** Topography of reflex zones (1).

▶ **Fig. 20.2** Topography of reflex zones (2).

ℹ Additional Information

Depending on whether a practitioner subscribes to one or the other school, localization of individual points varies significantly. This can be understood from the viewpoint that ear acupuncture points are in fact zones in which each active point may be localized.

21 Points on the Auricular Lobule According to Chinese Nomenclature

1 Analgesia Point for Tooth Extraction

Location: Quadrant I (▶ **Fig. 21.1**).

Indication: Analgesia for tooth extraction.

2 Roof of Mouth (Upper Palate)

Location: Quadrant II (▶ **Fig. 21.1**).

Indication: Trigeminal neuralgia, toothache.

3 Floor of Mouth (Lower Palate)

Location: Quadrant II (▶ **Fig. 21.1**).

Indication: Trigeminal neuralgia, toothache.

4 Tongue

Location: Quadrant II (▶ **Fig. 21.1**).

Indication: Stomatitis, toothache.

5 Upper Jaw

Location: Quadrant III (▶ **Fig. 21.1**).

Indication: Trigeminal neuralgia, toothache.

6 Lower Jaw

Location: Quadrant III (▶ **Fig. 21.1**).

Indication: Trigeminal neuralgia, toothache.

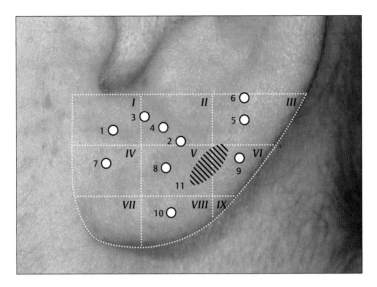

▶ **Fig. 21.1** Points on the lobule according to Chinese nomenclature.

7 Analgesia Point for Toothache

Location: Quadrant IV
(▶ Fig. 21.1).

Indication: Stomatitis, toothache.

8 Eye

Location: Quadrant V
(▶ Fig. 21.1).

Indication: Inflammatory eye disorders, hordeolum (stye), glaucoma, cephalgia that "radiates into the eyes."

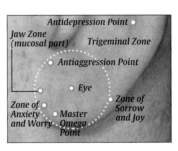

▶ **Fig. 21.2** Major points on the lobule according to Nogier.

9 Inner Ear

Location: Quadrant VI
(▶ Fig. 21.1).

Indication: Vertigo, tinnitus, hearing loss.

10 Tonsil

Location: Quadrant VIII
(▶ Fig. 21.1).

Indication: This point has lymphatic activity.

11 Cheek

Location: Quadrant V/VI
(▶ Fig. 21.1).

Indication: Facial paresis, trigeminal neuralgia.
   How to find the points: We can divide the lobule into nine fields by drawing three horizontal and two vertical lines and using the natural border of the ear lobe. This creates nine fields that contain the 11 acupuncture points of the lobule (▶ Fig. 21.1).
   For comparison: Important points on the lobule according to Nogier (▶ Fig. 21.2)
- Zone of Anxiety and Worry
- Zone of Sorrow and Joy
- Antidepression Point
- Antiaggression Point
- Master Omega Point
- Trigeminal Zone
- Maxillary sinus (mucous membrane components)

22 Points on the Auricular Lobule According to Nogier

Zone of Anxiety and Worry

Location: Anterior edge of the lobule, where it attaches to the head, at the level of the eye (▶ **Fig. 22.1**).

Indication: Anxiety (fear), worry.

> ❗ **Note**
> For right-handed patients:
> Anxiety (fear) is treated on the right ear (silver needle); worry is treated on the left ear (silver needle).
>
> For left-handed patients:
> Vice versa.

Antidepression Point

Location: On the extension of the vegetative groove, on a line that runs through Point Zero and C1. Correlates with localization of Point de Jérôme (▶ **Fig. 22.1**).

Indication: Depressive mood, psychosomatic disorders.

Antiaggression Point

Location: At the lower edge of the intertragic notch, toward the face (▶ **Fig. 22.1**).

Indication: Important psychotropic point. Addiction treatment.

Master Omega Point

Location: On the caudal part of the lobule, toward the face, on an imaginary line running vertically in front of the tragus peak (▶ **Fig. 22.1**).

Indication: Important psychotropic point; deep effect, vegetative harmonization.

Trigeminal Zone

Location: On the lateral edge of the ear, at the level of the antitragus and the lower cervical spine (▶ **Fig. 22.1**).

Indication: Trigeminal neuralgia.

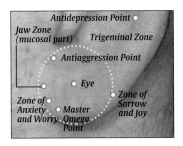

▶ **Fig. 22.1** Points on the lobule according to Nogier.

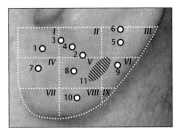

▶ **Fig. 22.2** Points on the lobule according to Chinese nomenclature.

Zone of Sorrow and Joy

Location: On the occipital part of the lobule, at the same level (▶ Fig. 22.1) as the zone of Anxiety and Worry.

Indication: Impaired joy of life, sorrow.

> **!** Note
>
> For right-handed patients: Impaired joy of life is treated on the right ear; sorrow is treated on the left ear.
>
> For left-handed patients: Vice versa.

Eye

Location: In the middle of the lobule (▶ Fig. 22.1).

Indication: Eye disorders, migraine, pollinosis.

Maxillary Sinus (Mucous Membrane Components)

Location: In the middle of the area of attachment of the lobule to the skin of the face (▶ Fig. 22.1).

Indication: Sinus disorders, interference field.

For comparison: Points on the lobule according to Chinese nomenclature (▶ Fig. 22.2)
- 1 Analgesia for Tooth Extraction
- 2 Roof of Mouth
- 3 Floor of Mouth
- 4 Tongue
- 5 Upper Jaw
- 6 Lower Jaw
- 7 Analgesia for Toothache
- 8 Eye
- 9 Inner Ear
- 10 Tonsil
- 11 Cheek

23 Points on the Tragus According to Chinese Nomenclature

12 Apex of Tragus

Location: On the cranial leg of a single-peaked tragus. On the cranial peak of a double-peaked tragus (▸ **Fig. 23.1**).

Indication: Analgesic, anti-inflammatory.

13 Adrenal Gland

Location: On the lower third of a single-peaked tragus. On the caudal peak of a double-peaked tragus (▸ **Fig. 23.1**).

Indication: Allergic diathesis, joint disorders, chronic inflammation, circulatory disorders, paresis, neuralgia.
  Generally indicated for all types of adrenal dysfunction.

14 External Nose

Location: In the middle of the base of the tragus (▸ **Fig. 23.1**).

Indication: Local disorders of the nose (eczema, rhinophyma, etc.).

15 Larynx/Pharynx

Location: On the inside of the tragus, at the level of Point 12 (▸ **Fig. 23.1**).

Indication: Pharyngitis, tonsillitis.

┌─ Caution ──────────────────
│ Danger of circulatory collapse (vagus irritation).
└───────────────────────────

16 Inner Nose

Location: On the inside of the tragus, at the level of Point 13 (▸ **Fig. 23.1**).

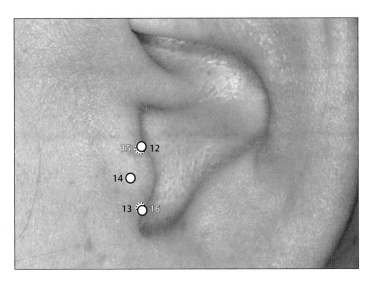

▶ **Fig. 23.1** Points on the tragus according to Chinese nomenclature.

Indication: Rhinitis, sinusitis.

┌─ Caution ─────────
│ Danger of circulatory col-
│ lapse (vagus irritation).

For comparison: Important points on the tragus and supra-tragic notch, according to Nogier and Bahr (▶ Fig. 23.2)

- Frustration Point
- Interferon Point
- Throat Point
- Laterality Point
- Valium Analogue Point
- Nicotine Analogue Point
- Pineal Gland Point

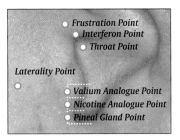

▶ **Fig. 23.2** Major points on the tragus and supratragic notch according to Nogier and Bahr.

24 Points on the Tragus According to Nogier and Bahr

Frustration Point

Location: In the groove between the tragus and crus of helix (▶ **Fig. 24.1**).

Indication: Psychosomatic disorders.

Interferon Point

Location: In the corner of the supratragic notch (▶ **Fig. 24.1**).

Indication: Immune-modulating effect, anti-inflammatory.

Throat Point

Location: In the cranioventral part of the inferior concha (▶ **Fig. 24.1**).

Indication: Disorders in the neck area, globus sensation, toothache.

Laterality Point

Location: On a horizontal line, approximately 3 cm from the middle of the tragus (▶ **Fig. 24.1**).

🔲 Note
Preferably perform needling in right-handed patients on the right side and (masked) left-handed patients on the left side.

Indication: Laterality dysfunction. This point strengthens inner balance through general stress relief. It provides inner (mental and emotional) stability for right–left oscillation, psychosomatic syndromes, and addiction treatment.

Valium Analogue Point

Location: On the descending part of the tragus (▶ **Fig. 24.1**; see also "How to Find the Points" [p. 161]).

Indication: Addiction treatment, general sedating effect.

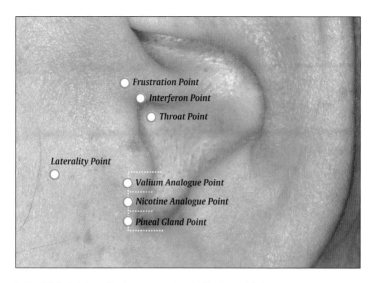

Frustration Point
Interferon Point
Throat Point
Laterality Point
Valium Analogue Point
Nicotine Analogue Point
Pineal Gland Point

▶ **Fig. 24.1** Points on the tragus according to Nogier and Bahr.

Nicotine Analogue Point

Location: Just below the Valium Analogue Point (▶ **Fig. 24.1**; see also "How to find the points" below).

Indication: Addiction treatment.

Pineal Gland Point

Location: Below the Nicotine Analogue Point (▶ **Fig. 24.1**; see also "How to find the points" below).

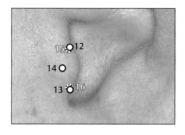

▶ **Fig. 24.2** Major points on the tragus according to Chinese nomenclature.

Indication: Functional psychotropic point; circadian rhythm disorders; supportive effect for hormonal disorders.

How to find the points: Draw a horizontal line through the middle of the tragus and another horizontal line through the bottom of the intertragic notch. Connect these two lines by drawing a vertical line approximately 3 mm in front of the tragus edge. Along this vertical line, divide the distance between the two horizontal lines into three sections. The following points are located in the middle of each section, from top to bottom: Valium Analogue Point, Nicotine Analogue Point, and Pineal Gland Point (▶ **Fig. 24.1**).

For comparison: Important points on the tragus according to Chinese nomenclature (▶ Fig. 24.2)

- 12 Apex of Tragus
- 13 Adrenal Gland
- 14 External Nose
- 15 Larynx/Pharynx
- 16 Inner Nose

25 Points on the Intertragic Notch According to Chinese Nomenclature

22 Endocrine Zone

Location: At the bottom of the intertragic notch, toward the face (▶ **Fig. 25.1**).

Indication: All endocrine disorders (gynecology, rheumatology, allergies, skin disorders).

🛈 **Additional Information**
According to Nogier, this zone corresponds to the points of the adrenal, thyroid, and parathyroid glands.

23 Ovary Point (Gonadotropin Point, According to Nogier)

Location: On the ventral and outer bulge (torus) of the antitragus ("Eye of the Snake" when viewing antitragus and anthelix as a snake) (▶ **Fig. 25.1**).

Indication: Ovarian dysfunction, period-related migraines and skin disorders.

24a Eye Point 1, 24b Eye Point 2

Location: Below the intertragic notch (▶ **Fig. 25.1**).

Indication: Non-inflammatory eye disorders, possibly myopia, astigmatism, optic nerve atrophy.

34 Gray Substance Point (Vegetative Point II, According to Nogier)

Location: On the inside of the antitragus, above the Ovary Point (▶ **Fig. 25.1**).

Indication: General balancing effect, antiphlogistic effect, analgesic affect.

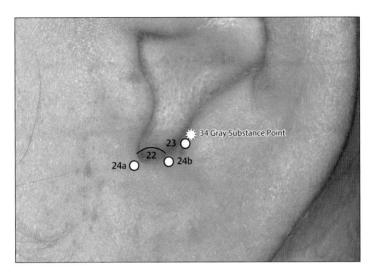

▶ **Fig. 25.1** Points on the intertragic notch according to Chinese nomenclature.

For comparison: Important points on the intertragic notch according to Nogier (▶ Fig. 25.2)

- ACTH Point
- Gonadotropin Point
- TSH (thyrotropin) Point
- Antiaggression Point
- Vegetative Point II

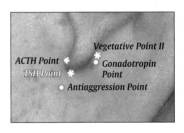

▶ **Fig. 25.2** Major points on the intertragic notch according to Nogier.

26 Points on the Intertragic Notch According to Nogier

ACTH Point

Location: On the caudal end to caudal third of the tragus, partly on the inside (▶ **Fig. 26.1**).

Indication: Important point for treatment of rheumatic disorders, bronchial asthma, skin disorders.

TSH Point

Location: In the middle of the intertragic notch, on the inside (▶ **Fig. 26.1**).

Indication: Thyroid gland disorders, urogenital tract disorders, skin disorders, bulimia.

Gonadotropin Point

Location: On the ventral and outer bulge (torus) of the antitragus ("Eye of the Snake" when viewing antitragus and anthelix as a snake) (▶ **Fig. 26.1**).

Indication: Sexual dysfunction, dysmenorrhea, amenorrhea.

Antiaggression Point

Location: At the lower edge of the intertragic notch, toward the face (▶ **Fig. 26.1**).

Indication: Important psychotropic point; addiction treatment.

Vegetative Point II (34 Gray Substance, According to Chinese Nomenclature)

Location: On the inside of the antitragus, at the caudal side.

Indication: Analgesic; vegetative balancing (harmonization).

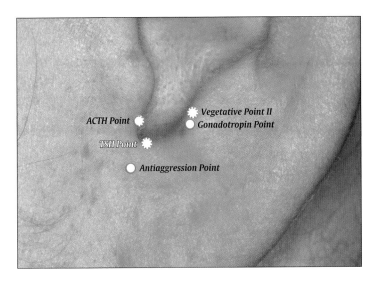

ACTH Point

TSH Point

Vegetative Point II
Gonadotropin Point

Antiaggression Point

▶ **Fig. 26.1** Points on the intertragic notch according to Nogier.

For comparison: Important points on the intertragic notch according to Chinese nomenclature (▶ Fig. 26.2)
- 22 Endocrine Zone
- 23 Ovary
- 24a Eye 1
- 24b Eye 2
- 34 Gray Substance

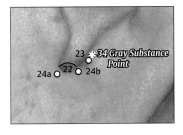

23   34 Gray Substance Point
24a   22   24b

▶ **Fig. 26.2** Major Points on the intertragic notch according to Chinese nomenclature.

27 Points on the Antitragus According to Chinese Nomenclature

26a Pituitary Gland (Thalamus, According to Nogier)

Location: On the inside of the antitragus, opposite Point 35 (▶ **Fig. 27.1**).

Indication: General analgesic point.

> ℹ **Additional Information**
> According to Nogier, effects the homolateral side of the body.

> ❗ **Note**
> Do not perform downward (descending) stimulation during pregnancy.

30 Parotid Gland

Location: On the tip of the antitragus (▶ **Fig. 27.1**).

Indication: Pruritus (strong antipruritic effect), inflammation of the parotid gland, mumps.

31 Asthma

Location: Between Points 30 and 33 (▶ **Fig. 27.1**).

Indication: Bronchitis, asthma; affects the respiratory center.

33 Forehead

Location: On the ventral part of the antitragus (▶ **Fig. 27.1**).

Indication: Disorders (-algia, -itis) in the forehead region; corresponds to the Frontal Bone Point according to Nogier; vertigo.

34 Gray Substance Point

Location: On the inside of the antitragus, above the gonadotropin point (▶ **Fig. 27.1**).

Indication: General balancing (harmonizing) effect, antiphlogistic effect, analgesic effect.

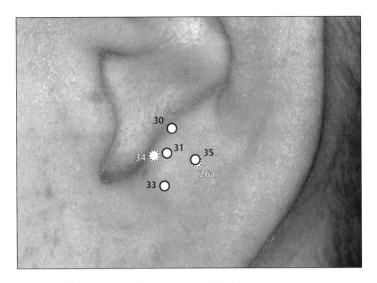

▶ **Fig. 27.1** Points on the antitragus according to Chinese nomenclature.

35 Sun

Location: In the middle of the base of the antitragus (▶ Fig. 27.1).

Indication: Very frequently used point. Cephalgia, migraine, eye disorders, vertigo, sleep disorders.

For comparison: Important points on the antitragus according to Nogier (▶ Fig. 27.2)

- Postantitragal Fossa
- 29 Occipital Bone
- 29a Kinetosis/Nausea Point
- 29b Jerome Point
- 29c Craving Point

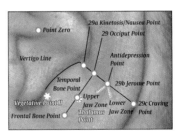

▶ **Fig. 27.2** Major points on the antitragus according to Nogier.

- Vertigo Line according to von Steinburg
- Vegetative II (Gray Substance)
- Thalamus
- Temporal Bone
- Frontal Bone
- Temporomandibular Joint

28 Points on the Antitragus According to Nogier

Postantitragal Fossa

Location: The Postantitragal Fossa is a straight line drawn from Point Zero through the notch between the antitragus and anthelix to the edge of the ear. Important acupuncture points (29a, 29b, 29c) are located on this line (▶ **Fig. 28.1**).

Indication: See Points 29a, 29, 29b, 29c.

29 Occipital Bone

Location: In the Postantitragal Fossa, approximately midway between Points 29a and 29b. According to Chinese nomenclature, the Occiput Point is localized slightly more toward the face (▶ **Fig. 28.1**).

Indication: Important analgesic point with a broad spectrum of activity. Conditions of pain, skin disorders, functional circulatory disorders, allergies, vertigo, autonomic dysfunction, convalescence.

29a Kinetosis/Nausea Point

Location: Between the anthelical edge and Point 29 (Occipital Bone; ▶ **Fig. 28.1**).

Indication: Kinetosis, vomiting.

29b Jerome Point
"Relaxation point"

(Multiple projection: Points 29b [Jerome Point], Temporomandibular Joint and Antidepression Point share the same projection area.)

Location: In the Postantitragal Fossa, at the intersection with the vegetative groove (▶ **Fig. 28.1**).

Indication: Vegetative harmonization. Difficulty falling asleep. In case of difficulty staying asleep, the corresponding point on the back of the ear is needled.

Temporomandibular Joint

Location: Jerome Point (▶ **Fig. 28.1**).

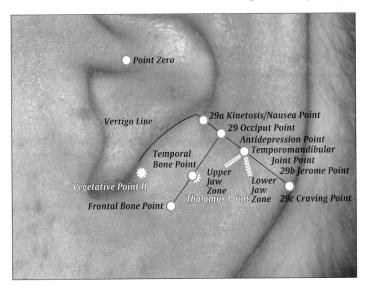

▶ **Fig. 28.1** Points on the antitragus according to Nogier.

There are several projection zones in the area of the Temporomandibular Joint:

- Palatine tonsil
- Molars of the upper and lower jaw
- Retromolar fossa (space)
- Posterior muscles of mastication
- Antidepression Point
- Magnesium Point (Bahr)
- Parotid Gland
- Insertion of lateral pterygoid muscle

Indications: Gnathologic problems, pain syndromes, tinnitus.

For comparison: Important points on the antitragus according to Chinese nomenclature (▶ Fig. 28.2)

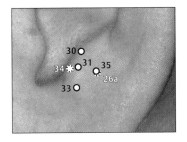

▶ **Fig. 28.2** Important points on the antitragus according to Chinese nomenclature.

- 26a Pituitary Gland
- 30 Parotid Gland
- 31 Asthma
- 33 Forehead
- 34 Gray Substance
- 35 Sun

Antidepression Point

Location: Jerome Point
(▶ Fig. 28.3).

Indications: Depressive mood, psychosomatic disorders.

29c Craving Point

Location: At the end of the Post-antitragal Fossa, at the intersection with the helical brim
(▶ Fig. 28.3).

Indication: Within the framework of addiction treatment.

Vertigo Line According to von Steinburg

Location: Runs along the Postantitragal Fossa and upper edge of the antitragus; slightly on the inside (▶ Fig. 28.3).

Indication: Vertigo.

Vegetative II (Gray Substance)

Location: On the inside of the antitragus, corresponds approximately to the Gray Substance Point (▶ Fig. 28.3).

Indication: Analgesic, vegetative harmonizing.

Thalamus Point (26a, Pituitary Gland, According to Chinese Nomenclature)

Location: On the inside of the antitragus, opposite the Temporal Bone Point (▶ Fig. 28.3; Point 35, Sun Point).

Indication: General analgesic point; vegetative harmonization. Premature ejaculation, female sexual dysfunction, influences the homolateral side of the body.

> **⚡ Practical Tip**
> In case of arthritis (rheumatism of the joints), use gold needles.

Temporal Bone Point (35, Sun Point, According to Chinese Nomenclature)

Location: In the middle of the base of the antitragus
(▶ Fig. 28.3).

Indication: Frequently used point. Cephalgia, migraine, eye disorders, vertigo, sleep disorders.

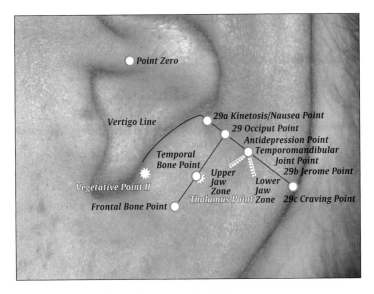

▶ **Fig. 28.3** Points on the antitragus according to Nogier.

Frontal Bone Point (33, Forehead According to Chinese Nomenclature)

Location: On the ventral part of the antitragus (▶ Fig. 28.3).

Indication: Disorders (-algia, -itis) in the area of the forehead.

For comparison: Important points on the antitragus according to Chinese nomenclature (▶ Fig. 28.4)

- 26a Pituitary Gland
- 30 Parotid Gland

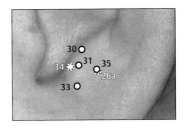

▶ **Fig. 28.4** Important points on the antitragus according to Chinese nomenclature.

- 31 Asthma
- 33 Forehead
- 34 Gray Substance
- 35 Sun

29 Projection of the Bony Skeleton According to Nogier

▶ Fig. 29.1

The cranial bones project on the area of the antitragus, with some multiple projections here, as with other areas. The frontal bone projects on the descending part of the antitragus. The ethmoid bone and the upper jaw project more toward the helical brim. The parietal bone projects on the tip of the antitragus. The projection of the occipital bone forms the border in the dorsal direction. The temporal bone projects in the middle of the antitragus. The temporomandibular joint, lower jaw, and teeth project next to the occipital bone.

The paranasal sinuses play a major role as interference fields. They also project in the antitragus region. The maxillary sinus projects in the area of the upper jaw. The frontal sinus lies slightly below the area of the frontal bone. The sphenoidal sinus and the ethmoidal sinuses project on a line in the immediate vicinity of the maxillary sinus.

The upper extremity has its projection zones in the area of the scapha, while the lower extremity projects in the triangular fossa.

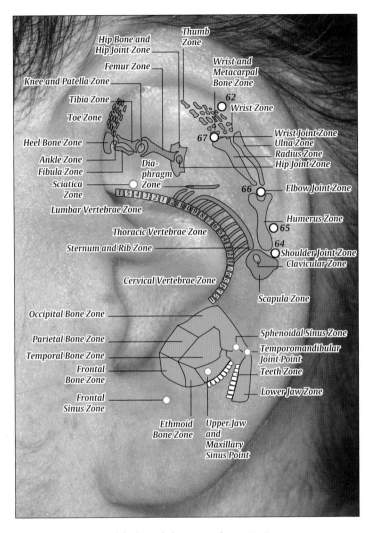

▶ **Fig. 29.1** Projection of the bony skeleton according to Nogier

30 Projection Zones of the Spinal Column According to Nogier

Nervous Organ Points of the Paravertebral Chain of Sympathetic Ganglia

C1/2 (▶ Fig. 30.1)

Location: Zone II. Superior Cervical Ganglion Point.

Indication: Tinnitus, vertigo.

C2/3 (▶ Fig. 30.1)

Location: Zone II. Middle Cervical Ganglion Point.

Indication: Functional heart disorders.

C7/T1 (▶ Fig. 30.1)

Location: Zone II. Inferior Cervical Ganglion Point, Stellate Ganglion Point.

Indication: Tinnitus, thoracodynia (chest pain); detecting interference fields.

Nervous Control Points of the Endocrine Glands

T12/L1 (Adrenal Glands, Location 1), T6 (Adrenal Glands, Location 2)

Different locations are listed according to the school to which they belong.

Location: Zone III. Adrenal cortex, cortisone point (▶ Fig. 30.1).

Indication: PCP (pneumocystis pneumonia in rheumatoid arthritis [RA]); allergies, general anti-inflammatory and analgesic effects.

T12 (Pancreas, Location 1), T6 (Pancreas, Location 2)

Different locations are listed according to the school to which they belong.

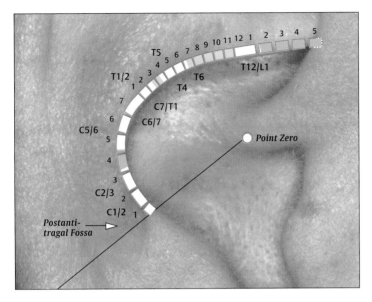

▶ **Fig. 30.1** Projection zones of the spinal column according to Nogier

Location: Zone III. Pancreas, insulin point (▶ Fig. 30.1).

Indication: Digestive disorders.

T4 (Thymus Gland, Location 1), T1/2 (Thymus Gland, Location 2)

Different locations are listed according to the school to which they belong.

Location: Zone III. Thymus (▶ Fig. 30.1).

Indication: Allergic disorders; effective against interference fields.

T5 (Mammary Gland)

(Also sometimes listed as a non-endocrine gland in this area [variation depending on school]).

Location: Zone III. Mammary (▶ Fig. 30.1).

Indication: Lactation disorders, premenstrual mastopathy.

C6/7 (Thyroid Gland)

Location: Zone III. Thyroid
(▶ **Fig. 30.1**).

Indication: Thyroid disorders,
globus sensation.

C5/6 (Parathyroid Gland)

Location: Zone III. Parathyroid
(▶ **Fig. 30.1**).

Indication: Bone disorders,
osteoporosis, fracture healing,
"cramps."

Cross-Section of Ear Relief (Zones I to VIII) (▶ Fig. 30.2)

I Zone of organ parenchyma
   II Zone of paravertebral chain of
sympathetic ganglia
   III Zone of nervous control
points of endocrine glands
   IV Zone of intervertebral disks
   V Zone of vertebrae
   VI Zone of paravertebral
muscles and ligaments
   VII Vegetative Groove (zone of
origin of sympathetic nuclei)
   VIII Zone of spinal cord with
projections of (a) motor tracts, (b)
autonomic tracts, (c) sensory
tracts

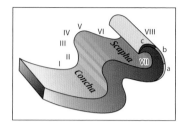

▶ **Fig. 30.2** Cross section of ear relief
(zones I to VIII).

31 Plexus Points in the Concha According to Nogier

Cardiac Plexus (Wonder Point)

Location: Ventral to the projection of the middle cervical ganglion, at the level of C2/3 (▶ Fig. 31.1).

Indication: Hypertension, functional heart problems.

Bronchopulmonary Plexus

Location: In the inferior concha, below the end point of the solar plexus (Oppression Point, ▶ Fig. 31.1).

Indication: Broncholytic effect.

Solar Plexus

Location: Zone including Point Zero and Oppression Point (▶ Fig. 31.1).

Indication: Gastrointestinal problems.

Hypogastric Plexus (Urogenital Plexus)

Location: On the upper edge of the crus of helix, toward the superior concha, approximately in the middle between Point Zero and the intersection of the ascending helix and inferior anthelical crus. Identical with Omega Point 1 (▶ Fig. 31.1).

Indication: Gastrointestinal and urogenital problems, renal colic.

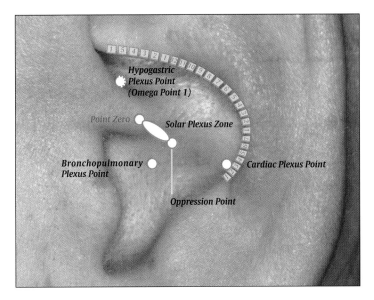

▶ **Fig. 31.1** Plexus points in the concha according to Nogier.

For comparison: Projection zones of internal organs according to Nogier (▶ Fig. 31.2**)**

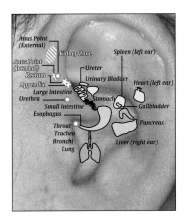

▶ **Fig. 31.2** Projection zones of internal organs according to Nogier.

32 Points in the Triangular Fossa According to Chinese Nomenclature

49 Knee Joint

Location: In the middle of the superior anthelical crus (▶ **Fig. 32.1**).

Indication: Pain in the knee area —more related to functional disorders.

❗ Note
The "French" Knee Point is located in the middle of the triangular fossa and represents rather an anatomy projection of the knee joint.

51 Autonomic (Sympathetic Point, Vegetative Point I)

Location: At the intersection of the inferior anthelical crus and helix (▶ **Fig. 32.1**).

Indication: An important acupuncture point. Vegetative harmonization, vegetative balancing of all visceral organs.

55 Shen Men "Divine Gate"

Location: Above the angle formed by the superior and inferior anthelical crura, more toward the superior anthelical crus (▶ **Fig. 32.1**).

Indication: One of the most important ear acupuncture points.
Strong mental and emotional balancing effect; functional point for conditions of pain; anti-inflammatory.

56 Pelvis

Location: In the angle formed by the superior and inferior anthelical crura (▶ **Fig. 32.1**).

Indication: Pain in the pelvic area.

ℹ Additional Information
Hip Point and Pelvis Point according to Nogier are identical with Point 56.

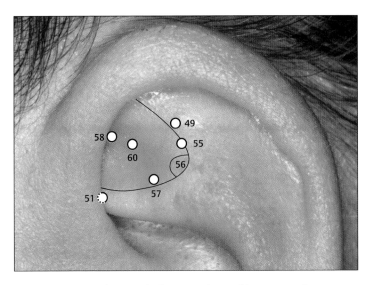

▶ **Fig. 32.1** Points in the triangular fossa according to Chinese nomenclature.

57 Hip

Location: At the lower margin of the triangular fossa, ventral to Pelvis Point 56 (▶ Fig. 32.1).

Indication: Pain in the hip region.

58 Uterus

Location: In the triangular fossa, close to the helix (▶ Fig. 32.1).

Indication: Conditions after uterus extirpation (total hysterectomy), for example, postoperative pain.

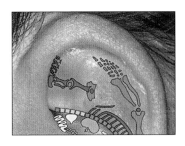

▶ **Fig. 32.2** Projection zones in the triangular fossa according to Nogier.

60 Dyspnea

Location: Lateral (and caudal) to Uterus Point 58 (▶ Fig. 32.1).

Indication: Bronchial asthma.
  For comparison: Projection zones in the triangular fossa according to Nogier (▶ Fig. 32.2)

33 Points on the Ascending Helix According to Chinese Nomenclature

78 Apex of Ear (Allergy Point According to Nogier)

Location: At the tip of the ear, formed by folding the auricula (helix margin in the direction of crus of helix) (▶ **Fig. 33.1**).

Indication: General immune-modulating effect—for example, allergies, bronchial asthma.

79 External Genitals

Location: On the ascending helix, at the level of the intersection with the inferior anthelical crus (▶ **Fig. 33.1**).

Indication: All forms of erectile dysfunction; migraine, dysuria.

80 Urethra

Location: At the level of the intersection of the ascending helix and lower edge of the inferior anthelical crus (▶ **Fig. 33.1**).

Indication: Urinary tract infection, dysuria.

82 Diaphragm

Location: On the ascending helix, cranioventral to the crus of helix, in a distinctly palpable fossula; topographic location corresponds to Nogier's Point Zero (▶ **Fig. 33.1**).

Indication: Hematological disorders, spasmolytic effect.

> **ℹ Additional Information**
> According to Nogier, this is *the* classic point of energy control.

83 Bifurcation Point

Location: At the origin of the crus of helix (▶ **Fig. 33.1**).

Indication: The Chinese school does not assign any major significance to this point.

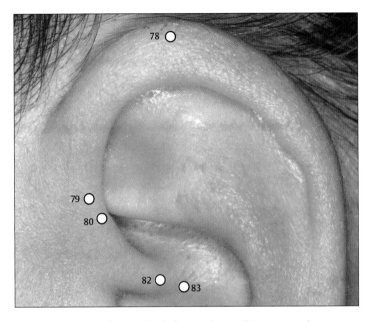

▶ **Fig. 33.1** Points on the ascending helix according to Chinese nomenclature.

ℹ Additional Information
According to Nogier, this is the end point of the solar plexus (Oppression Point).

⚡ Practical Tip
Often, this point is needled for states of anxiety. Also called "Anxiety Point 2."

For comparison: Important points on the ascending helix according to Nogier (▶ Fig. 33.2)
- Point R
- External Genitals
- (External) Anus

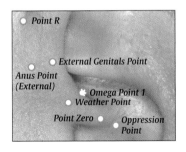

▶ **Fig. 33.2** Important points on the ascending helix according to Nogier.

- Omega 1
- Point Zero
- Oppression Point
- Weather Point

34 Points on the Helix According to Nogier

Omega 2

Location: On the upper edge of the helix, ventral to Allergy Point 78, at the tip of the ear (▶ Fig. 34.1).

Indication: Important functional regulating point for motor function; point for disturbed relationship with the environment.

Point R (R. J. Bourdiol)

Location: On the extension of the ascending helix, in the fossula at the transition to facial skin (▶ Fig. 34.1).

Indication: Adjuvant point in psychotherapy.

External Genitals

Location: On the ascending helix, at the level of the inferior anthelical crus (▶ Fig. 34.1).

Indication: All forms of erectile dysfunction, migraine, dysuria.

(External) Anus

Location: On the helix brim, approximately at the intersection of the extension of the inferior anthelical crus (▶ Fig. 34.1).

Indication: Anal problems, anal pruritus.

Omega 1

Location: At the upper edge of the crus of helix, in the inferior concha, approximately in the middle between Point Zero and the intersection of the ascending helix and inferior anthelical crus (▶ Fig. 34.1).

Indication: Metabolic disorders, vegetative disorders, mercury exposure.

Weather Point (Kropej)

Location: In the middle of a line between the supratragic notch and the intersection of the inferior anthelical crus and helix (▶ Fig. 34.1).

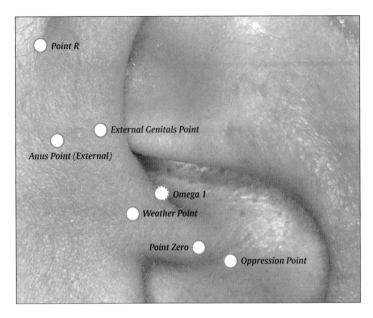

▶ **Fig. 34.1** Points on the helix according to Nogier.

Indication: Sensitivity to changes in the weather (meteoropathy, atmosphere related syndrome, ARS); adjuvant point for angina pectoris and migraine, often detectable on the right ear.

🔲 **Practical Tip**
Relative contraindication in case of pregnancy.

For comparison: Important points on the helix according to Chinese nomenclature (▶ Fig. 34.2)

- 78 Apex of the Ear (Allergy Point according to Nogier)

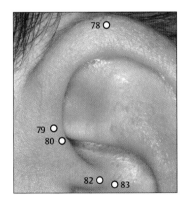

▶ **Fig. 34.2** Important points on the helix according to Chinese nomenclature.

- 79 External Genitals
- 80 Urethra
- 82 Diaphragm
- 83 Bifurcation

Point Zero

Location: On the ascending helix, cranioventral to the crus of helix, in a distinctly palpable fossula; topographic location corresponds to Point 82 (Diaphragm) in Chinese localization (▶ **Fig. 34.1**).

Indication: According to Nogier, this is *the* classic point of energy control.

> ⚡ **Practical Tip**
>
> Treatment with gold needles for psychovegetative exhaustion; treatment with silver needles in case of excessive needle reaction.

Furthermore, Point Zero has a strong spasmolytic effect.

78 Allergy Point

Location: At the tip of the ear, formed by folding the auricula (margin of helix in the direction of crus of helix) (▶ **Fig. 34.2**).

Indication: General immune-modulating effect—for example, allergies, bronchial asthma.

Oppression Point

Location: At the origin of the crus of helix (end point of the Solar Plexus), corresponding to Point 83 (Bifurcation Point) in the Chinese school (▶ **Fig. 34.1**).

Indication: According to Nogier, the end point of the Solar Plexus. Also called Anxiety Point, which reflects its indication: state of anxiety, functional gastrointestinal disorders.

35 Covered Points on the Helix According to Nogier

Gestagen Point

Location: Close to the fold of the ascending helix, on the inside, at the level of the superior anthelical crus (▶ **Fig. 35.1**).

Indication: Hormonal imbalance, hormone-related migraine.

Renin–Angiotensin Point

Location: Above the Renal Parenchyma zone, on the inside (▶ **Fig. 35.1**).

Indication: Arterial hypertension (silver needle on right ear), hypotension (gold needle on right ear).

Renal Parenchyma Zone

Location: On the inside of the helix, approximately at the level of the triangular fossa (▶ **Fig. 35.1**).

Indication: Kidney disorders.

Hemorrhoid Point (Coccygeal Bone Point)

Location: On the end of the inferior anthelical crus (covered by helix) (▶ **Fig. 35.1**).

Indication: Hemorrhoidal problems, pain in the coccygeal region (coccydynia).

Uterus

Location: Approximately at the intersection of the superior anthelical crus and the helix, on the inside (▶ **Fig. 35.1**).

Indication: Dysmenorrhea, interference field after hysterectomy.

> **Practical Tip**
> Acupuncture of points on the ascending helix is contraindicated during pregnancy.

Prostate

Location: Between Ovary/Testis Point and Uterus Point, on the inside (▶ **Fig. 35.1**).

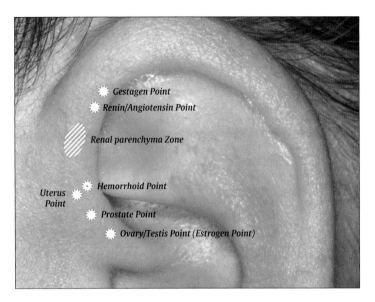

▶ **Fig. 35.1** Covered points on the helix according to Nogier.

Indication: Prostatitis, prostate interference field.

Ovary/Testis (Estrogen Point)

Location: Slightly above the supra-tragic notch, inside the ascending helix, approximately 2 mm away from the reflection (▶ **Fig. 35.1**).

Indication: Hormonal dysfunction, hormone-related migraine.

For comparison: Important points on the helix according to Chinese nomenclature (▶ Fig. 35.2)

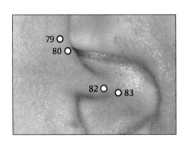

▶ **Fig. 35.2** Important points on the helix according to Chinese nomenclature.

- 79 External Genitals Point
- 80 Urethra Point
- 82 Diaphragm Point
- 83 Bifurcation Point

36 Projection Zones of Internal Organs According to Chinese Nomenclature

84 Mouth

Location: Upper part of the supratragic notch (▶ **Fig. 36.1**).

Indication: Trigeminal neuralgia, stomatitis.

85 Esophagus

Location: Below the middle of the ascending crus of helix (▶ **Fig. 36.1**).

Indication: Problems in the esophageal region.

86 Cardiac

Location: Lateral to the Esophagus Zone 85 (▶ **Fig. 36.1**).

Indication: Stomach problems, reflux.

87 Stomach

Location: Surrounding the crus of helix (▶ **Fig. 36.1**).

Indication: Stomach problems, gastritis, ulcer, nausea, vomiting.

88 Duodenum

Location: Superior concha, above the crus of helix (▶ **Fig. 36.1**).

Indication: Gastrointestinal problems.

89 Small Intestine

Location: In the superior concha, adjacent to Duodenum Zone 88 (▶ **Fig. 36.1**).

Indication: Gastrointestinal problems.

90 Appendix Zone 4

Location: Ventral adjacent to the Small Intestine Zone 89 (▶ **Fig. 36.1**).

Indication: This point has a lymphatic effect.

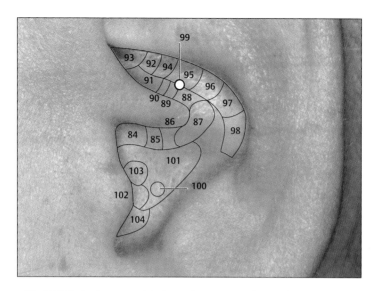

▶ **Fig. 36.1** Projection zones of the internal organs according to Chinese nomenclature.

91 Large Intestine

Location: In the superior concha, opposite Zone 94 (▶ Fig. 36.1).

Indication: Gastrointestinal complaints, meteorism, obstipation, diarrhea.

92 Urinary Bladder

Location: Cranial to Zone 91 (▶ Fig. 36.1).

Indication: Urogenital tract disorders, dysuria, incontinence.

For comparison: Projection zones of internal organs according to Nogier (▶ Fig. 36.2)

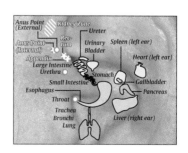

▶ **Fig. 36.2** Projection zones of the internal organs according to Nogier.

93 Prostate

Location: On the floor of the superior concha, in the angle formed by the ascending helix and inferior anthelical crus (▶ **Fig. 36.1**).

Indication: Prostate disorders, dysuria, erectile dysfunction.

94 Ureter

Location: Lateral to Zone 92 (▶ **Fig. 36.1**).

Indication: Dysuria.

> 🔲 **Practical Tip**
> Often used in combination with the Kidney Zone 95.

95 Kidney

Location: In the middle of the cranial part of the superior concha (▶ **Fig. 36.1**).

Indication: This is one of the most important zones in ear acupuncture. It is used for urogenital tract disorders as well as for joint disorders, menstrual problems, migraine, sleep disorders, functional problems and disorders of the ear, and for addiction treatment.

These points (▶ **Fig. 36.1**) do not have a fixed location, but are located in a zone. Needling takes place at the most sensitive point.

> 🔲 **Practical Tip**
> These points are needled according to their "meaning."

> ┌─ Caution ───────────
> Be careful when needling points near the external acoustic meatus (danger of vasovagal dysregulation).

96 Pancreas and Gallbladder

Location: Next to Zone 95 (▶ **Fig. 36.3**).

ⓘ Additional Information
According to Chinese localization, the gallbladder projects on the right ear and the pancreas on the left ear. According to Nogier, the head of the pancreas also projects on the right ear, while the body and tail of the pancreas project on the left ear.

Indication: Cholecystopathy, digestive disorders.

97 Liver

Location: At the transition of the superior and inferior concha, lateral to the Stomach Zone 87, near the anthelix (▶ **Fig. 36.3**).

ⓘ Additional Information
On the right ear, the liver projects in Zones 97 and 98. In the left ear, the liver projects in Zone 97.

Indication: Gastrointestinal disorders, hematological disorders, skin disorders, eye disorders. An important zone within the scope of addiction treatment.

98 Spleen

Location: Caudal to Zone 97, in the inferior concha, close to the anthelix (▶ **Fig. 36.3**).

ⓘ Additional Information
In the right ear, the liver projects in Zones 97 and 98. In the left ear, the liver projects in Zone 97.

Indication: Digestive disorders, hematological disorders.

99 Ascites Point

Location: Between zones 88, 89, and 95 (▶ **Fig. 36.3**).

Indication: An adjuvant point in liver disorders.

100 Heart

Location: In the middle of the inferior concha (▶ **Fig. 36.3**).

Indication: Psychovegetative dysregulation, hypertension, hypotension, sleep disorders, anxiety, heart problems, depression.

101 Lung

Location: Surrounding Zone 100
(▶ **Fig. 36.3**).

Indication: Respiratory tract disorders, skin disorders. Used within the scope of addiction treatment, especially during nicotine withdrawal.

102 Bronchus

Location: Medial to the Lung Zone, toward the external meatus (▶ **Fig. 36.3**).

Indication: Respiratory tract disorders.

103 Trachea

Location: Above Zone 102
(▶ **Fig. 36.3**).

Indication: Respiratory tract disorders.

104 Triple Energizer

Location: Below Zone 102
(▶ **Fig. 36.3**).

Indication: An adjuvant point for hormonal disorders.

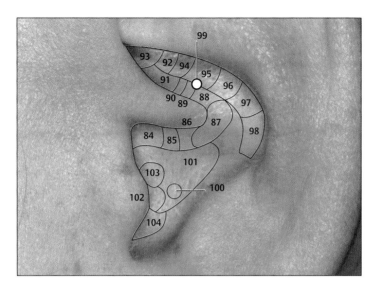

▶ **Fig. 36.3** Projection zones of the internal organs according to Chinese nomenclature.

For comparison: Projection zones of the internal organs according to Nogier (▶ Fig. 36.4)

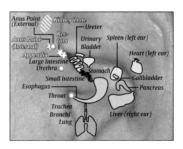

▶ **Fig. 36.4** Projection zones of the internal organs according to Nogier.

37 Projection Zones of Internal Organs According to Nogier

The organs of the upper half of the body project to the inferior concha. The organs of the lower half of the body project to the superior concha. Exceptions: The heart projects to the anthelix and the kidney and genital organs project to the ascending helix (▶ Fig. 37.1).

> **!** Note
> Blood and lymph vessels always project near the structures they supply.

Heart

Location: On the anthelix, at the level of T4 to T7, left ear (▶ Fig. 37.1).

Indication: Supportive effect for pumping function.

Lung

Location: In the middle of the inferior concha (▶ Fig. 37.1).

Indication: Respiratory tract disorders.

Bronchus

Location: Cranial to the lung zone, toward the supratragic notch (▶ Fig. 37.1).

Indication: Respiratory tract disorders.

Trachea

Location: Medial cranial to the bronchial projection zone (▶ Fig. 37.1).

Indication: Respiratory tract disorders.

Throat

Location: On the floor of the cavity of the concha, in the area of the supratragic notch (▶ Fig. 37.1).

Indication: Respiratory and throat disorders, addiction therapy.

Esophagus

Location: Below the crus of helix; toward the face, tapering off into the Throat Zone (▶ **Fig. 37.1**).

Indication: Disorders in the area of the esophagus.

Stomach

Location: Half-moon shaped, around the crus of helix (▶ **Fig. 37.1**).

Indication: Stomach disorders.

Duodenum

Location: Adjacent to the Stomach Zone, in a cranial direction (▶ **Fig. 37.1**).

Indication: Stomach and duodenum disorders.

Small Intestine

Location: Lower and middle part of the superior concha (▶ **Fig. 37.1**).

Indication: Gastrointestinal tract disorders.

Large Intestine

Location: Upper part of the superior concha (▶ **Fig. 37.1**).

Indication: Gastrointestinal tract disorders.

Appendix

Location: Posterior to the ascending helix, in the angle it forms with the concha, at the medial margin of the superior concha (▶ **Fig. 37.1**).

Indication: This is frequently an interference zone and can be treated via the ear.

Rectum

Location: Under the ascending helix, in the anterior medial (not visible) part of the superior concha (▶ **Fig. 37.1**).

Indication: Gastrointestinal tract disorders.

Anus

Location: Inner mucous membrane component: on the inferior anthelical crus, below the crus of helix (▶ **Fig. 37.1**).

Indication: Anal disorders, hemorrhoids.

Liver

Location: Right ear, in the lateral and middle part of the concha (▶ **Fig. 37.1**).

Indication: Liver dysfunction, supportive for hepatitis.

Gallbladder

Location: Middle third of the superior concha (▶ **Fig. 37.1**).

Indication: Gallbladder disorders, migraine.

Pancreas

Location: Caudal to the Gallbladder Zone, in the superior concha (▶ **Fig. 37.1**).
   The "endocrine part" of the pancreas projects to the anthelix at the level of T12.

Indication: Pancreas disorders.

Spleen

Location: Left ear, in the superior concha, cranial to the Pancreas Zone (▶ **Fig. 37.1**).

Indication: Hematological disorders, digestive disorders.

Kidney Zone

Location: Covered, below the helix, at the level of the middle of the triangular fossa (▶ **Fig. 37.1**).

Indication: Kidney disorders.

Ureter

Location: Medial adjacent to the Bladder Zone, in the concha (▶ **Fig. 37.1**).

Indication: Disorders of the ureter.

Bladder

Location: In the superior concha, at the projection of the upper lumbar spine (▶ **Fig. 37.1**).

Indication: Bladder disorders.

Urethra

Location: At the anterior margin of the ascending helix, where the cartilage margin is palpable (▶ **Fig. 37.1**).

Indication: Urethra disorders.

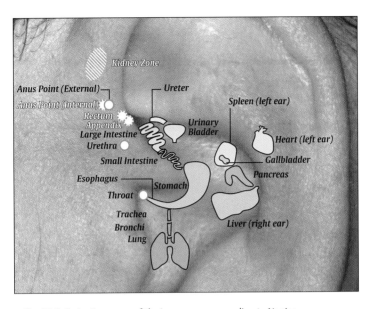

▶ **Fig. 37.1** Projection zones of the inner organs according to Nogier.

For comparison: Projection zones of the internal organs according to Chinese nomenclature (▶ Fig. 37.2)

- 84 Mouth
- 85 Esophagus
- 86 Cardia
- 87 Stomach
- 88 Duodenum
- 89 Small Intestine
- 90 Appendix 4
- 91 Large Intestine
- 92 Urinary Bladder
- 93 Prostate
- 94 Ureter
- 95 Kidney
- 96 Pancreas and Gallbladder
- 97 Liver
- 98 Spleen
- 99 Ascites

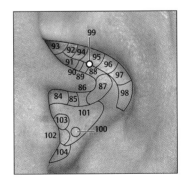

▶ **Fig. 37.2** Projection zones of the inner organs according to Chinese nomenclature.

- 100 Heart
- 101 Lung
- 102 Bronchial
- 103 Trachea
- 104 Triple Energizer

38 Energy and Treatment Lines on the Auricula

Several energy lines and treatment lines have been described on the auricula. Active acupuncture points are frequently found along these treatment lines (▶ Fig. 38.1). They usually form a basic framework for designing individual treatment schemes.

Postantitragal Fossa

Location: The postantitragal fossa is a straight line from Point Zero through the notch between the antitragus and anthelix to the edge of the ear (▶ Fig. 38.1). Important acupuncture points (29a, 29, 29b, 29c) are located on this line.

29a Kinetosis/Nausea Point

Location: At the transition of the antitragus to the anthelix, between Point 25 (Brain Stem Point, on the edge of the anthelix, at the transition of the antitragus to the anthelix) and Point 29 (Occiput Point) (▶ Fig. 38.1).

Indication: Nausea, vomiting, and motion sickness.

29 Occiput Point

Location: In the postantitragal fossa, approximately midway between the Kinetosis/Nausea Point 29a and Jerome Point 29b (▶ Fig. 38.1).

Indication: Important analgesic point, especially for cephalgia.

29b Jerome Point (Relaxation Point)

Location: In the postantitragal fossa, at the intersection with the vegetative groove (▶ Fig. 38.1).

Indication: Important point with vegetative harmonizing effect for psychosomatic disorders and sexual dysfunction; sleep disorders.

> 🔧 **Practical Tip**
>
> According to Nogier, needling of Point 29b is performed with a gold needle for difficulty in falling asleep. A silver needle is preferred for difficulty in staying asleep.

29c Craving Point

Location: At the end of the post-antitragal fossa, on the helical brim (▶ **Fig. 38.1**).

Indication: Psychosomatic disorders, addiction treatment.

Sensory Line

Nogier calls the line between the Frontal Bone Point (33, Forehead Point), Temporal Bone Point (35, Sun Point), and Occipital Bone Point (29, Occiput Point) the Sensory Line. This line is associated with energetic blood flow to the head, similar to the body acupuncture points PdM (Point de Merveille) and GV-16 (▶ **Fig. 38.1**).

The postantitragal fossa and the Sensory Line represent two basic pillars for treatment by ear acupuncture. The respective conspicuous points may be used together with the related spinal-column segment for basic therapy in treatment of pain.

Stress Furrow

Location: The stress furrow is a fold that runs diagonally across the auricular lobule. We find it often in patients who are under stress or cannot cope with stress in an appropriate manner. This furrow is of purely diagnostic importance (▶ **Fig. 38.1**). It has no therapeutic application.

Vegetative Groove

Location: The vegetative groove runs cranially from the postanti-tragal fossa below the helical brim to the intersection of the inferior anthelical crus and ascending helix (▶ **Fig. 38.1**).

Indication: The vegetative groove represents an important treatment element in ear acupuncture. It should be examined for active points prior to each treatment.

Line of Omega Points

This is the line connecting the three Omega Points according to Nogier. It runs vertically in front of the tragus tip (▶ **Fig. 38.1**).

Nogier divides the ear into three zones:
- The Endodermal Zone is assigned to metabolism
- The Mesodermal Zone is assigned to motor function
- The Ectodermal Zone is assigned to the head and central nervous system and,

therefore, to a higher level of regulation

Corresponding to this tripartition, Nogier found a control point for each zone.

Omega 2

Location: On the upper edge of the helix, on the nasal side of Allergy Point 78, on an imaginary line running vertically in front of the tragus tip (▶ **Fig. 38.1**).

Sphere of action: Mesodermal Zone; innervated by the auriculo-temporal nerve of the trigeminal nerve.

Assignment: Motor function. A point for disturbed relationships with the environment.

Omega 1

Location: On the upper edge of the crus of helix, approximately in the middle of a line from Point Zero and the intersection of the ascending helix and inferior anthelical crus, on an imaginary line running vertically in front of the tragus tip (▶ **Fig. 38.1**).

Sphere of action: Endodermal Zone; innervated by the vagus nerve.

Assignment: Metabolism.

Master Omega Point

Location: On the ventral lower part of the lobule, on an imaginary line running vertically in front of the tragus tip (▶ **Fig. 38.1**).

Sphere of action: Ectodermal Zone; innervated by the cervical plexus.

Assignment: Head and central nervous system.

Vertigo Line According to von Steinburg

Location: Runs along the postantitragal fossa and on the inside of the antitragus; it is used in case of vertigo (▶ **Fig. 38.1**).

Indication: Vertigo.

Needle method: Search for the most reactive point or points on this line.

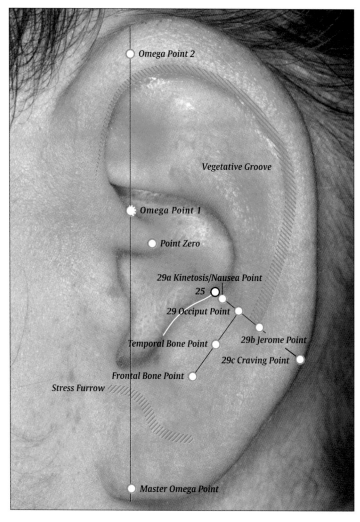

Omega Point 2

Vegetative Groove

Omega Point 1

Point Zero

29a Kinetosis/Nausea Point
25
29 Occiput Point

Temporal Bone Point

29b Jerome Point

29c Craving Point

Frontal Bone Point

Stress Furrow

Master Omega Point

▶ **Fig. 38.1** Energy and treatment lines on the auricula.

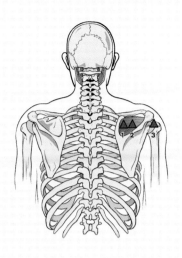

Part 3
Trigger Points

39 Definition of Trigger Points

The term "myofascial trigger point" (MTrP) was coined by D. J. Simons and J. Travell in the 1950s. Trigger points refer to local, circumscribed hardenings in muscles. These are painful on palpation (pressure sensitive) and cause a sensation of pain at a distance from the source (referred pain). Trigger points are characterized by a local twitch response of the muscle during needling or infiltration of the trigger point area. Frequently, this phenomenon can be readily induced by deep palpation of the trigger point area. A trigger point is caused by the contraction of sarcomeres in a muscle fiber. A contraction knot or disk formed by several muscle fibers is relatively easy to palpate (▶ Fig. 39.1). The remaining parts of the muscle fiber become stretched and form a hard muscle band (taut band) that is also easy to palpate. Chronic trigger points show a histological change in the Z disks. Electromyography (EMG) reveals an increased electrical activity in the trigger point region without detecting alpha motor neuron (α-motoneuron) activity.

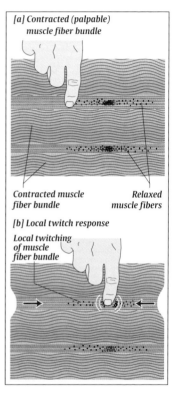

[a] Contracted (palpable) muscle fiber bundle

Contracted muscle fiber bundle

Relaxed muscle fibers

[b] Local twitch response

Local twitching of muscle fiber bundle

▶ Fig. 39.1 Diagram of a trigger point complex.

Epidemiology

According to studies by Raspe, the lifetime prevalence of back pain in Germany is more than 80%.[104] Point prevalence, that is, back pain experienced at the time of surveying, is expected to be about 35%.[103]

More than half of all treatments performed by orthopedic specialists and 25% of treatments by general practitioners are for back pain.[103] Studies further show that 25% of all low back pain patients cause about 95% of the expenditure for musculoskeletal disorders.[139] In the United States, the total expenses for musculoskeletal disorders are expected to amount to 1% of the gross national product.[141] In Germany, total costs for disability due to back pain were 17 billion euros in 1998.[17]

It would be wrong to assume that the diverse symptoms experienced by patients are caused by severe structural problems. On the contrary, these persistent symptoms are often induced by ordinary muscle tension in combination with poor posture and secondary dysfunction of joint movements. Conventional treatment with medication and physiotherapy often ends in frustration for both patients and therapists. Spontaneous healing rates for acute myofascial pain syndromes are high (more than 90%), but relapse rates are also extremely high. As a result, recurrent dysfunctions often develop into chronic myofascial pain syndromes.

Muscle Physiology

Basic tension in the muscular system is directly coupled with activity of the sympathetic nervous system. Increased sympathetic activity always causes muscle hypertonicity.[84] Relaxed muscles show no electrical activity on the electromyograph (EMG).[9]

It is important to distinguish between viscoelastic tone and contractile activity.[85] Viscoelastic tone is influenced by the sliding of myofibrils toward each other[31] and it declines during major movements.[138] Most changes in muscle tone exhibit a change in electrical activity. Muscle tone is regulated by gamma motor neurons (γ-neurons). Stretch receptors in the muscle spindles respond to changes in length with a monosynaptic reflex; stretching therefore induces an increased activity of alpha motor neurons. During contraction or at rest, afferent signals from the muscle spindles are not expected. Afferent signals from the gamma motor neurons stimulate small intrafusal muscle fibers within the muscle spindle and cause the muscle spindle to contract. This increases muscle tone. To protect muscles from traumatic rupture, special stretch receptors in the Golgi tendon organs are stimulated during rapid passive stretching or intense active contraction of the muscle. The resulting reflex inhibition of alpha motor neurons leads to a reduction in muscle tone.

A number of factors can change resting muscle tone. Pain affects the tone of the surrounding muscles. If the cause of pain is in the muscle itself, the alpha motor neurons show no electrical activity. However, pain resulting from segmental reflexes, such as visceral pain or arthrogenic pain, often leads to increased tone in the surrounding muscles (▸ Fig. 39.2).[86]

Emotional tension also increases muscle tone that is often restricted to certain regions of the shoulder girdle.[83] Climate factors, such as cold and humidity, can also increase muscle tone.[133]

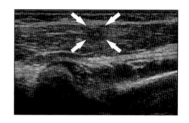

▸ **Fig. 39.2** Ultrasound visualization of a trigger point in the long radial extensor muscle of the wrist.

Pathophysiology of Myofascial Pain

Myofascial pain syndromes usually start with single or repetitive muscle strain, such as acute overstretching or, in rare cases, in response to a direct traumatizing blow to a specific muscle region.[8,122] Myofascial pain syndromes are often found in patients who perform repetitive, usually monotonous arm and hand movements while maintaining unfavorable body posture.[4,79] Among those most impacted are musicians,[27,112] people working at computers,[53] industrial and assembly-line workers,[3,121] but also athletes for whom repetitive movements cause problems.[25,40]

Muscle contraction is triggered by an action potential in the motor neurons of the anterior horn cells. The action potential causes the opening of ion channels in the presynaptic membrane of the neuromuscular junction (motor endplate) and an influx of Ca^{++} ions into the nerve terminals. This results in the release of acetylcholine into the synaptic cleft, which in turn leads to the opening of ion channels in the postsynaptic membrane of the muscle fiber and to the creation of a new action potential that now spreads across the entire surface of the muscle fiber. The smallest contractile unit is the

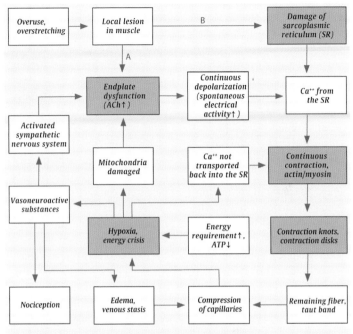

Dejung 1999 (adapted after Simons, Mense, Dommerholt, Gröbli)

▶ **Fig. 39.3** Pathophysiology of myofascial pain syndrome.

sarcomere, where actin molecules and myosin heads slide against each other. This requires the presence of the energy carrier ATP. Releasing the myosin heads from the actin filaments requires a lot of energy. With insufficient ATP, the myosin heads cannot release from the actin and thus form a rigor complex. According to the energy crisis theory, persistent rigor complexes at certain muscle sites are the pathophysiological basis of myofascial dysfunction.[122]

The energy crisis theory, in combination with the results of histological and electromyographical studies on trigger points, provides the best explanation for the observed phenomena. However, a definitive explanation is currently not possible. Findings to date show that the motor endplate hypothesis preferred by Simons does not provide a complete explanation and requires additional studies. Development of a myofascial pain syndrome is always based on acute or chronic overuse or overstretching of the affected muscle (▶ Fig. 39.3). Theoretically, two different patterns of injury are possible:

- First, a dysfunction of the endplate leads to a continuous release of small amounts of acetylcholine into the synaptic cleft. The alpha motor neuron shows no action potential. The release of acetylcholine causes persistent depolarization of the postsynaptic membrane of the muscle fiber. This action potential registers as spontaneous electrical activity of the endplate.[52]

- Second, according to more recent observations, a local muscle lesion may cause traumatic damage of the sarcoplasmic reticulum and thus increased release of Ca^{++} ions. In this context, a certain distance between endplate and contraction disk, or contraction knot, has been observed.[99] Pongratz favors this phenomenon as the cause of subsequent pathophysiological processes.

The developing action potential travels on the membrane of the muscle fiber in all directions and reaches the sarcoplasmic reticulum inside the muscle fiber via the transverse tubules (T tubules). This results in a persistent release of Ca^{++} ions.

Also discussed, as a pathophysiological cause of trigger point formation, is a leak in the sarcoplasmic reticulum. The resulting damaged endplate or damaged calcium ion compartment causes persistent contracture of the sarcomeres. This consumes large quantities of calcium and ATP. A significant aggregation of contracted sarcomeres creates contraction knots or disks. The sum of these contraction disks and knots of a muscle fiber then results in a palpable trigger point. The remaining affected muscle fibers are stretched and form a palpable taut band. Overstretching of the affected muscle fibers causes strangulation of capillaries and ischemia of the entire muscle region. Depletion of ATP in the presence of increased ATP demand causes an energy crisis of the muscle section involved. This is reinforced by hypoxia, with a drop in partial oxygen pressure toward zero in the trigger point. Hypoxia damages the mitochondria, which increases dysfunction of the endplate. This lack of energy prevents the detachment of actin and myosin filaments and creates a rigor complex (▸ Fig. 39.4).

Hypoxemia and energy crisis of the muscle cause the release of vasoneuroactive substances, such as bradykinin, serotonin, histamine, and substance P. This results in hyperemia in the region surrounding the trigger point. Increased vascular permeability creates local edema with reactive venous stasis and influx congestion in the arterioles. This further increases ischemia within the trigger point. The transition from aerobic to anaerobic metabolism causes acidosis in the tissue, which in turn sensitizes and stimulates the muscle nociceptors (▸ Fig. 39.5). Release of vasoneuroactive substances results in activation of the sympathetic nervous system. This increased sympathetic activity leads to increased release of acetylcholine at the endplate and thus further potentiates the dysfunction of the endplate.

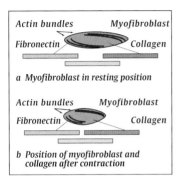

a Myofibroblast in resting position

b Position of myofibroblast and collagen after contraction

▸ **Fig. 39.4** Connective tissue structures newly formed during repair phase begin to contract after two weeks under the influence of myofibroblasts.

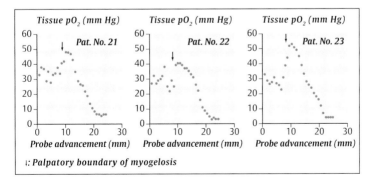

ᵢ: Palpatory boundary of myogelosis

▸ **Fig. 39.5** Tissue pO₂ measurement in tense back muscles.

These pathological mechanisms are further amplified by factors resulting from the patient's individual condition: Lack of exercise, together with insufficient capillarization of the muscles and poor formation of mitochondria, promote this vicious cycle. Essentially, all factors that increase muscle tone lead to strangulation of the capillaries. Myogelosis, in turn, can damage motor nerve function and, therefore, directly negatively impact endplate function.[16]

Other research results also support the integrated hypothesis for the development of trigger points.

A working group led by Kuan[72] discussed the spinal cord connections of the myofascial trigger spots. No differences were shown compared to afferent and efferent nerve fibers of uninvolved muscles. However, the motor neurons of trigger point muscle fibers were smaller in diameter.

Results presented by Shah et al,[118,119] show a significant increase of inflammatory tissue mediators and a decrease in tissue pH using microdialysis when compared to uninvolved muscles. These results are yet to be confirmed.

Recently, treatment of the fascia has gained increased attention, especially also from an osteopathic approach to therapy. According to Paoletti,[92] fasciae are the basic connective tissue structures that interconnect all organ systems. There are fascial structures, especially in muscles, that contain contractile elements. Since the body tries to achieve optimal economy, muscles with primarily postural (static support) function are equipped with thick fasciae. These fasciae are able to receive muscle tension and to maintain the desired state of tension (tone). This makes it possible for the body to maintain static postures over long periods with the least possible use of energy.[92,117]

Chronic myogelosis of muscles containing trigger points leads to a restructuring of fascia and muscles and hardening (contracture) of connective tissue. This has considerable therapeutic consequences. In addition to loosening restrictions usually present in the joint region through manual manipulation or treating only the trigger points, fascial contractions need to be treated at the same time.[50,108]

Chronification Model of Myofascial Pain Syndromes

Treatment of acute trigger points in the context of short-term overuse injury usually does not pose a problem. After treatment of the trigger points, symptoms will completely disappear. Chronic myofascial pain syndromes, however, pose considerable therapeutic challenges. Peripheral sensitization at the trigger point has already been described.[106] Continuous influx of nociceptive signals at the posterior horn leads to a transformation in terms of a wind-up of spinal cord neurons. This reorientation of interneurons, in turn, leads to sensitization of the first or second projection neuron in the posterior horn. The wide-dynamic range neuron (WDR neuron) sends nociceptive signals to the thalamus via the ascending pathway in the anterior spinothalamic tract. Here, signal transmission occurs via the internal capsule and external capsule into the limbic system and from there to the cerebral cortex. Regrouping takes place also in the cerebral system, with a change in the projection zones of the affected muscles (or body regions) and with over-representation causing a change in the mind map. Frequently, a disturbance develops in the descending inhibitory pain system. It is through these mechanisms that an originally peripheral nociceptive disorder develops from a primarily segmental disorder into a regional disorder, and finally into a systemic pain disorder. This condition considerably interferes with daily life because the patient undergoes changes in pain perception and frequently also develops unfavorable coping strategies. Integration of this disorder into a biopsychosocial disease model[29] is not only difficult for the patient but also for the physician, who often gives in to the patient's concept of disease, which emphasizes the typical cause-and-effect pattern ("treat the location of the problem to fix it").

Another consideration is that unfavorable coping strategies, such as a sense of helplessness and hopelessness[42] and dissatisfaction in the workplace[29] are important predictors for unfavorable treatment outcomes. It is therefore essential that trigger point therapy is part of a multimodal therapeutic concept to address myofascial pain disorders, as these can soon become chronic.

Basic Therapeutic Considerations

In order to treat trigger points appropriately, the affected muscle must be classified within the myofascial tension system. This system was described by Richardson, Jull et al in 1999.[106] In this system, the deep internal muscle layer represents the osteoligamental structure that is essential for segmental stability. The superficial external layer is formed by mostly long, multiarticular muscles that function primarily as motor muscles. Between these two layers is a layer of muscles responsible for balance and active segmental stability.

Examples of the *deep layer* are local muscles like those of the spine: rotator muscles, multifidus muscles, long muscle of the neck and rectus capitis muscles. Those of the upper limbs include the infraspinatus and supraspinatus muscles, the subscapular muscle and the teres minor muscle. Those of the lower limbs include the vastus medialis muscle and the popliteal muscle. Examples of the *intermediate layer* are the obliquus externus muscle, the multifidi muscles, the deltoid muscle, and the vastus lateralis, intermedius, and medialis muscles. Examples of globally functioning and multiarticular muscles of the *superficial layer* are the rectus abdominis muscle, the sternocleidomastoid muscle, the scalene muscles, the trapezius muscle, the latissimus dorsi muscle, the biceps muscle of arm (long head), the rectus femoris muscle, and the biceps muscle of the thigh.

The clinical relevance of this subdivision is obvious. Strengthening these local muscles is highly recommended for preventing segmental instabilities. Studies have demonstrated its long-term effect in the context of rehabilitation programs for reduction of recurring pain.[49] Discomfort in local muscles is very often associated with musculoskeletal problems.[66,91]

Dysfunctions of multiarticular muscles are frequently associated with acute musculoskeletal problems, but less often with chronic problems.[51,56] Frequently, there is premature activity associated with innervation. This muscle type tends toward muscular atrophy, with extreme reduction in muscular circumference. By comparison, local muscles tend to show a reduction in type I fibers, with clear reductions in capillary and fiber circumference and increased fat and connective tissue components.

Clinical examination of this group of muscles involves voluntary selective submaximal tension. In the case of global monoarticular muscles, muscle function tests are performed for strength, endurance, and muscle balance, whereas global multiarticular muscles are examined using stretch sensitivity tests, provocation, muscular balance, and by testing the neural structures.

Specific Trigger Point Examination and Basic Therapy Considerations

The most important diagnostic tool is to consider the possibility of trigger points in the first place. Trigger points are indicated by characteristic problems of the patient, whereby the overlapping projection zones of different trigger points make high demands on the therapist's knowledge of anatomy and physiology.

The DGS-Practice Questionnaire for Therapy of Spine, Back, Shoulder and Neck Pain, introduced by Überall et al[135] provides a test that facilitates the diagnosis of myofascial symptoms. Trigger points are frequently located in the center of muscle bellies. Considering osteopathic principles and based on clinical experience, it can be said that myofascial trigger points are found in agonists as well as in antagonists. Osteopathy differentiates between stretched hypertonic and contracted hypertonic muscles. Using the example of finger flexors and finger extensors, the following can serve to illustrate the difference between stretched hypertonic and contracted hypertonic muscles in a way that is relevant to daily practice. This primarily applies to multiarticular agonistic and antagonistic muscles, for example, the lower arm muscles, where making a fist requires simultaneous contraction of finger flexors and extensors, viz. the flexor muscles are contracted whereas the extensors are overstretched. If the finger flexors in particular are persistently contracted, these muscles will develop latent—that is, non-active—trigger points. Patients will rarely complain about radiating problems in

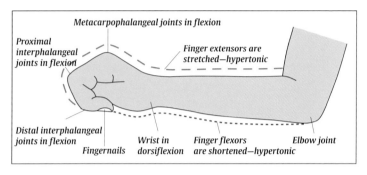

Metacarpophalangeal joints in flexion

Proximal interphalangeal joints in flexion

Finger extensors are stretched—hypertonic

Distal interphalangeal joints in flexion

Fingernails

Wrist in dorsiflexion

Finger flexors are shortened—hypertonic

Elbow joint

▶ **Fig. 39.6** Illustration of contracted finger flexor and stretched finger extensor.

their hands in the sense of referred pain. When palpated, these trigger points in particular will also exhibit local twitch responses. Clinical experience has shown, however, that with stretched hypertonic muscles (in this case the common extensor muscle of the fingers), taut bands can occur and palpable trigger points can develop in the muscle bellies of these relatively weak muscles (compared to finger flexors). This can give rise to radiating pain along the lower arm to the hands. Shortened hypertonic muscles are created by neuronal overstimulation, either from excessive exercise or from irritation of the nerve fibers supplying the muscle. These nerve irritations can be caused by nerve root

irritation or nerve compression (entrapment neuropathy).

Identifying and differentiating these differences in muscle tonicity is key for therapeutic success. It makes sense that the deactivation of trigger points in stretched hypertonic muscles can only bring short-lived success, because it does not resolve the underlying causative problem of muscular imbalance of the shortened hypertonic muscles. Durable deactivation of the trigger points in the area of the stretched hypertonic muscles requires treatment of the shortened muscles—for example, by stretching—as well as treatment of the underlying processes that cause the muscles to contract (▶ Fig. 39.6).

Clinical examination involves monodigital palpation or bidigital palpation using index finger and thumb (pinch grip) to provide orientation for the muscle in question. A local twitch response of the muscle can often be provoked in the trigger point area, and this response is accompanied by a characteristic radiation of pain into the projection zones of the trigger point. Frequently, corresponding satellite trigger points are also present and these should also be treated.

Meanwhile, myofascial trigger points can be diagnosed using ultrasound and magnetic resonance imaging (MRI) technology. Ultrasound elastography can identify palpable contraction nodules in a taut band. Studies by Sikdar et al,[120] based on work by Taylor et al[128] and confirmed by Turo et al,[134] primarily used vibration sonoelastography (combination of external vibration source with Doppler or duplex ultrasound). These studies showed trigger points as focal, elliptically configured, mostly hypoechoic zones that correlate with palpable local muscle hardening. Differentiation of surrounding nodules was also possible. There was no significant difference in size between active and latent trigger points. There was a notable presence of small arteries or enlarged arterioles near MTrPs in duplex ultrasound that showed retrograde flow in diastole, indicating a highly resistive vascular bed. These local changes were not seen in control groups without MTrPs.

High resolution 3-Tesla MRI can show structures in a very small field of view in high resolution and with very good soft tissue contrast. The skin above trigger points is marked with nitroglycerine capsules. These markers are easily visible in the MRI sequences and enable positive image-morphological correlation with the underlying palpable trigger points, which exhibit well-defined, rounded signal modifications within the muscle in the MR image. The T2-weighted sequences showed near isointensity in the center compared with the surrounding muscles. The surrounding area was delineated by a hypointense and a somewhat less focused hyperintense border. Some of these indurations were chevron shaped. Increased numbers of vessels with hemostasis were confirmed with morphological MRI. The stiffness of the palpable taut band was 9.0 kPa, which exceeded that of uninvolved muscles by 50%.[21]

There are many options for the treatment of trigger points. Dry-needling is the most effective method.[41] It involves insertion of an acupuncture needle directly into the contraction knot and fan-like manipulation of the needle in order to trigger local twitch responses. These responses are induced as long as necessary to deactivate the trigger point, which can be confirmed by palpation once the contraction knot has dissolved. Dry-needling is followed by targeted stretching of the muscle. The stretching techniques should be demonstrated to the patient and suggested as home exercise in order to prevent relapses.

With chronic tension, fascial therapy using the techniques of manual medicine is essential. Joint dysfunctions, which are a source of relapses for trigger points, should also be treated using manual techniques.

Wet-needling, that is, therapeutic injection of a local anesthetic, is usually not required and does not offer any advantage over dry-needling, because its effect is not derived from the local anesthetic.[86] Other therapeutic methods, such as myofascial release, acupoint massage (acupressure) combined with ischemic compression, or punctate transcutaneous electrical nerve stimulation (PuTENS), may be employed.[26] Electrotherapies or the use of TENS (transcutaneous electrical nerve stimulation) are less suitable. TENS, nevertheless, is of high value in the context of general pain management of myofascial pain syndromes.

40 Temporal Muscle

Description of the Muscle

▶ Fig. 40.1

Origin: Deep lamina of temporal fascia, temporal plane, temporal fascia of sphenoid bone, back of zygomatic bone.

Insertion: Coronoid process of the mandible, at its medial surface toward the third molar.

Innervation: Deep temporal nerves from the mandibular nerve (mandibular division of trigeminal nerve, third division of fifth cranial nerve).

Action: Raises lower jaw; posterior part: retrusion, supports mastication (chewing) movements.

Note: The superficial temporal artery runs on top of the muscle; it splits into parietal and frontal branches in the temporal area.

Trigger Points

Introduction: The temporal muscle has four trigger point areas (▶ Fig. 40.2) which can be located on an imaginary line running toward the ear, beginning at the inferior part of the muscle at the level of the lateral corner of the eye.

These trigger points are activated by malocclusion, direct traumas or longer-term immobilization, but also by dental procedures or psychogenic factors (e.g., bruxism or clenching of the teeth) and less often by external climatic factors such as draft or cold. Also to be considered are trigger points in the ipsilateral masseter muscle and in the contralateral temporal muscle. The medial and lateral pterygoid muscles, either unilaterally or bilaterally, are involved less often. Satellite trigger points appear as painful zones in the upper parts of the trapezius muscle and sternocleidomastoid muscle.

A differential diagnosis should consider temporal arteritis, polymyalgia rheumatica, and polymyositis. However, the typical pain projection areas which characterize trigger points are absent in these conditions.

Examination of trigger points:
Palpate the trigger point regions with the patient's mouth opened approximately 2 cm and the head stationary. Identify local, pressure-sensitive indurations of the muscle with typical pain projection. Palpate the inside of the mandibular coronoid process intraorally. Identify taut bands in the muscles where a brief local twitch response of the muscle can be triggered.

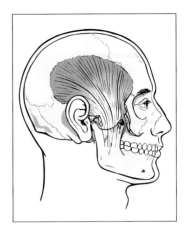

▶ **Fig. 40.1** Temporal muscle.

Trigger point therapy: While avoiding both branches of the temporal artery, the trigger points are needled conventionally, with the needles remaining in place for 20 minutes. Alternatively, the shortened muscles can be relaxed directly by intramuscular stimulation with the acupuncture needles. Trigger point infiltration with a local anesthetic in low concentration may also be considered. This is followed by passive stretching of the muscle by pulling the lower jaw down and forward, and using postisometric relaxation if indicated.

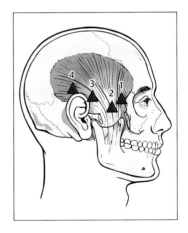

▶ **Fig. 40.2** Trigger points of the temporal muscle.

Trigger Points and Pain Projection Areas

Trigger point 1: Located in the anterior part of the muscle (▶ **Fig. 40.3**) and exhibits the following pain projection areas: incisors of the upper jaw, lateral lower wing of the nose, eyebrow, and anterior part of the temporal bone.

Trigger point 2: Located in the anterior portion of the medial part of the muscle (▶ **Fig. 40.4**). Radiating symptoms are found in the region of the canine tooth and first premolar of the upper jaw. Additional pain projections are located cranial to the trigger point.

Trigger point 3: Located in front of the auricula (▶ **Fig. 40.5**). Pain projection areas are located in the molar region of the upper jaw, and also along the middle fibers of the temporal muscle above the trigger point zone.

Trigger point 4: Located behind the auricula (▶ **Fig. 40.6**). Pain projection area dorsally along the fibers of the temporal muscle.

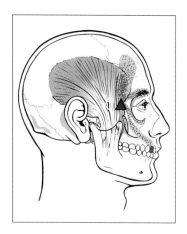

▶ **Fig. 40.3** Temporal muscle, trigger point 1.

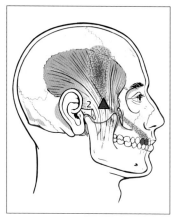

▶ **Fig. 40.4** Temporal muscle, trigger point 2.

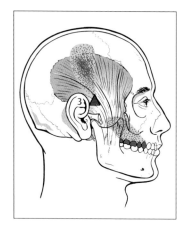

▶ **Fig. 40.5** Temporal muscle, trigger point 3.

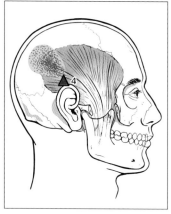

▶ **Fig. 40.6** Temporal muscle, trigger point 4.

Important Acupuncture Points

► Fig. 40.7, ► Fig. 40.8

ST-8

Location: 0.5 Cun from the frontal hairline toward the hair, in the angle of this hairline with the temporal hairline running perpendicular to it. This point is located 4.5 Cun lateral to GV-24.

EX-HN-5 (Extra 5, Tai Yang)

Location: Approximately 1 Cun toward the ear from the center of the line connecting the end of the eyebrow with the lateral corner of the eye.

ST-7

Location: In the center of the depression below the zygomatic arch, that is, in the mandibular notch between the coronoid process and condylar process of the mandible.

The mandibular condyle can be easily palpated in front of the tragus (it slips forward when opening the mouth). ST-7 is located in the depression just in front of it. This point is searched for and needled when the mouth is closed.

TE-22

Location: At the level of the auricular insertion, slightly ventral and cranial to TE-21, dorsal to the superficial temporal artery.

GB-8

Location: 1.5 Cun above the highest point of the auricula.

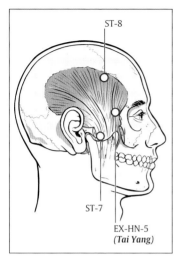

▶ **Fig. 40.7** ST-8, EX-HN-5, and ST-7.

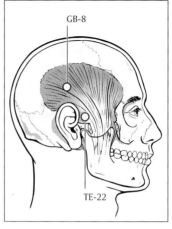

▶ **Fig. 40.8** TE-22 and GB-8.

Gnathologic Aspects

Temporal Muscle, Anterior Part

▶ Fig. 40.9

Functional aspects: Adductor muscle (closes the mouth).

Palpation: About 1 cm behind the lateral orbital margin.

Symptomatology: Parietal headache, central clenching of teeth, near-central grinding of teeth.

Projected pain:
- Pain in the medial and lateral incisors of the upper jaw (pulpal symptoms, hypersensitivity, prolonged pain response to thermal stimuli), sometimes sensation of pre-contact
- Toward the temple
- From the temple through the upper jaw bone toward the incisors of the upper jaw
- In a parietal direction
- In a supraorbital direction
- In a retrobulbar direction

Temporal Muscle, Medial Part

▶ Fig. 40.9

Functional aspects:
- Adductor muscle (closes the mouth) with the medial part only

- Retractor together with the posterior part

Palpation: Cranial to the ear.

Symptomatology:
- Temporal headache
- Occipital headache

Parafunction:
- Protrusion
- Retrusion

Projected pain:
- Into the larynx
- Toward the temple
- From the temple through the lateral upper jaw and zygomatic arch toward the canine tooth and first premolar of the upper jaw; pain in the area of the canine tooth and first premolar of the upper jaw (pulpal symptoms, hypersensitivity, prolonged pain response to thermal stimuli), sometimes sensation of pre-contact

Temporal Muscle, Posterior Part

▶ Fig. 40.9

Functional aspects:
- Adductor (closes the mouth) together with the medial part
- Retractor when supported by the medial part

Palpation: Cranial to the ear.

Symptomatology:
- Temporal headache
- Occipital headache

Parafunction:
- Protrusion
- Retrusion
- Contributes to the displacement of the condyles with secondary dysfunctions of the articular disk (dislocation of disk)

Projected pain:
- Into the larynx
- Toward the temple
- From the temple through the zygomatic arch into the lateral upper jaw; into the mucosa and into the molars; pain in the area of the second premolar and molars of the upper jaw (pulpal symptoms, hypersensitivity, prolonged pain response to thermal stimuli); sometimes sensation of pre-contact

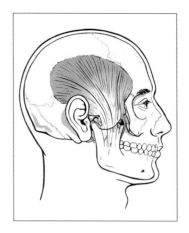

▶ **Fig. 40.9** Gnathologic aspects of the temporal muscle.

41 Masseter Muscle

▶ Fig. 41.1

Description of the Muscle

Origin:
- Superficial part: lower border of the lateral surface and temporal process of the zygomatic bone
- Deep part: lower border of the medial surface of the zygomatic arch

Insertion:
- Superficial part: angle of the mandible, toward the region of the second molars
- Deep part: toward the upper third of the ramus of the mandible (masseteric tuberosity) and toward the base of the coronoid process

Innervation: Deep temporal nerves from the mandibular nerve (mandibular division of trigeminal nerve).

Action: Raises the lower jaw, supports protrusion.

Note: At the anterior margin of this muscle, the facial artery crosses the edge of the mandible.

Trigger Points

Introduction: The masseter muscle encompasses seven trigger points: six in the superficial part and only one in the deeper portion of the muscle. These trigger points may be activated by bruxism, psychogenic factors, temporomandibular joint dysfunction (e.g., as a result of malocclusion), missing teeth, or jaw movement dysfunction resulting from tooth displacement. Trigger points may also be activated by acute traumas and acute strain. Frequently, these trigger points are activated through primary trigger points in the sternocleidomastoid muscle. Secondary trigger points are located in the temporal muscle and medial pterygoid muscle and less often in the contralateral masseter muscle.

Examination of trigger points: With the mouth opened approximately 2 cm, examine trigger point regions by pressing on the trigger point zones while providing intraoral support. The typical projected pain can be triggered, and taut bands can be palpated within the muscle.

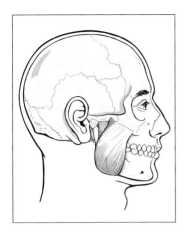

▶ **Fig. 41.1** Masseter muscle.

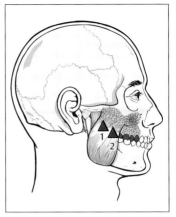

▶ **Fig. 41.2** Masseter muscle, trigger points 1 and 2.

Trigger point therapy: These trigger points are needled in the conventional way, with the needles remaining in place for 20 minutes. Taut bands can be released in a targeted way using intramuscular stimulation. If necessary, trigger point infiltration with a local anesthetic is also possible. Then follows passive stretching of the muscle by pulling the upper jaw down and forward, which patients can continue on their own.

Trigger Points and Pain Projection Areas

Trigger points 1 and 2: Located in the superficial part of the muscle at the level of the upper-jaw teeth (▶ Fig. 41.2). Pain is projected into molars and premolars as well as into the upper jaw.

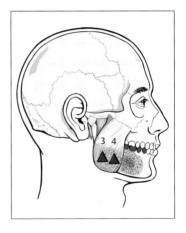

▶ **Fig. 41.3** Masseter muscle, trigger points 3 and 4.

Confusion with maxillary sinusitis is possible.

Trigger points 3 and 4: Located at the level of the mandibular center (▶ Fig. 41.3). Pain is projected into the lower jaw in front of the masseter muscle and into the region of the premolars and molars of the lower jaw.

Trigger points 5 and 6: Located at the insertion of the superficial portion (▶ Fig. 41.4). Pain projection areas are the lower jaw bone, the eyebrow, and, facultatively, the region between mandibular angle and ipsilateral eyebrow.

Trigger point 7: Located immediately in front of the temporomandibular joint in the deep portion of the masseter muscle (▶ Fig. 41.5). Pain is localized over the temporomandibular joint and in the region of the inferior concha of the ear. Diffused pain may also be present over the entire region of the masseter muscle.

Important Acupuncture Points

▶ Fig. 41.6

ST-5

Location: Ventral to the mandibular angle at the anterior margin of the masseter muscle. Pulsation of the facial artery can be palpated here.

ST-6

Location: Starting from the mandibular angle approximately 1 Cun ventral and in craniofacial direction. The masseter muscle can be palpated here when biting down.

ST-7

Location: In the center of the depression below the zygomatic arch, that is, in the mandibular notch between the coronoid process and condylar process of the mandible. The condylar process of the mandible can be easily palpated in front of the tragus (it slides forward when opening the mouth). ST-7 is located in the depression immediately in front of it.

SI-18

Location: At the lower edge of the zygomatic arch, vertically below the outer corner of the eye, at the anterior margin of the masseter muscle.

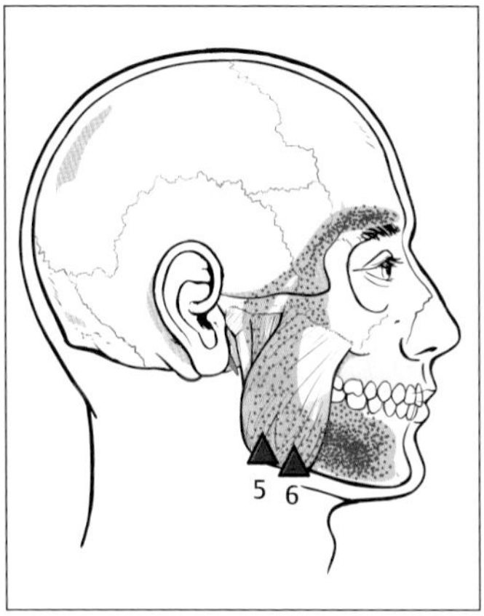

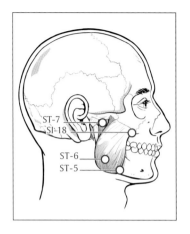

▶ **Fig. 41.4** Masseter muscle, trigger points 5 and 6.

▶ **Fig. 41.6** ST-5, ST-6, ST-7, and SI-18.

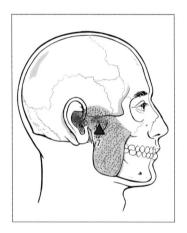

▶ **Fig. 41.5** Masseter muscle, trigger point 7.

Gnathologic Aspects

Masseter Muscle, Superficial Part

▶ Fig. 41.7

Functional aspects: Adductor muscle (closes the mouth), protractor muscle:
- Supports mediotrusion when contracted on one side
- Supports protrusion when contracted on both sides

Palpation: During relaxed state and when maximally contracted:
- At the origin below the zygomatic arch within the muscle belly
- With two fingers at the insertion with mouth open, 1 cm cranial to the angle of the mandible at the aponeurosis
- With both hands at the dorsal part of the body of the mandible

Symptomatology: In case of severe pain: trismus (inability to open the mouth normally), bruxism, mainly in the protruding position
- at the canine tooth if the muscle is shortened on one side, and
- at the edge of the incisors if the muscle is shortened on both sides

Projected pain: From the area of the premaxilla in a retrobulbar direction and into the maxillary sinus (sinusitis-like symptoms), into the distribution areas of the infraorbital nerve and maxillary division of the trigeminal nerve; in general, the upper jaw (in the bone) and mucosa of the lateral upper jaw.

Trigger point in the cranial part: Pain in the second premolar, first and second molars of the upper jaw (pulpal symptoms, hypersensitivity, prolonged pain response to thermal stimuli).

Trigger point in the medial part: Pain in the second premolar, first and second molars of the lower jaw (pulpal symptoms, hypersensitivity, prolonged pain response to thermal stimuli); pain in the lower jaw in the region of the molars.

Trigger point in the lower part: Pain radiating across the zygomatic arch and the anterior temporal area in a suborbital direction toward the entire eyebrow and supraorbital arch; in rare cases: unilateral tinnitus.

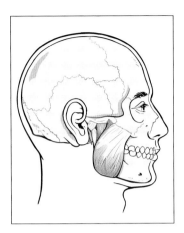

▶ **Fig. 41.7** Gnathologic aspects of the masseter muscle, superficial part.

42   Lateral Pterygoid Muscle

Description of the Muscle

▶ Fig. 42.1

Origin:
- Superior head: infratemporal fascia and infratemporal crest of greater wing of sphenoid bone
- Inferior head: lateral surface of lateral pterygoid plate of sphenoid bone
- Caudal head: between the two heads of the medial pterygoid muscle

Insertion: Upper edge of the pterygoid pit of the mandible, joint capsule and intra-articular disc of the temporomandibular joint.

Innervation: Lateral pterygoid nerve from the mandibular nerve (mandibular division of trigeminal nerve).

Action: Lowers mandible, causes mandible to protrude, moves mandible from side to side.

Trigger Points

Introduction: This two-bellied muscle contains two trigger points which rarely manifest due to acute events (e.g., traumas), but usually as a result of chronic strain of the temporomandibular joint with malocclusion and psychosomatic disorders (e.g., bruxism). Trigger points in this region rarely appear alone, but rather in combination with trigger points of the masseter muscle and of posterior fibers of the temporal muscle.

Examination of trigger points: With the mouth opened approximately 3 cm, palpate the muscle part close to the mandibular joint, between the joint and zygomatic bone; with the mouth opened 5 to 8 mm and starting from the cheek, palpate the muscle parts located further from the joint, above the coronoid process of the mandible.

Trigger point therapy: The following therapies may be considered: dry-needling, conventional acupuncture, and therapeutic local anesthesia. Reaching the muscle requires precise anatomical knowledge. The trigger points are at a depth of 3 cm. Stretching the muscle is usually only possible through physiotherapeutic mobilization of the temporomandibular joint.

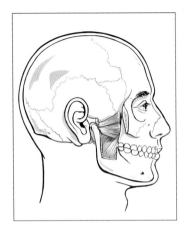

▶ **Fig. 42.1** Lateral pterygoid muscle.

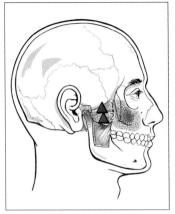

▶ **Fig. 42.2** Lateral pterygoid muscle, trigger points 1 and 2.

Trigger Points and Pain Projection Areas

Trigger points 1 and 2: The trigger point in the cranial part of the muscle (1) is located below the zygomatic arch, the other one (2) below the coronoid process of the mandible (▶ **Fig. 42.2**). The typical projection areas are located over the temporomandibular joint and at the level of the zygomatic arch.

Important Acupuncture Point
ST-7

Location: In the center of the depression below the zygomatic arch, that is, in the mandibular

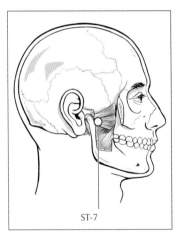

ST-7

▶ **Fig. 42.3** ST-7.

notch between the coronoid process and condylar process of the mandible (▶ **Fig. 42.3**).

Gnathologic Aspects

(▶ Fig. 42.4)

Functional aspects: Bilateral activity, abductor. Unilateral activity, mediotrusion.

   Palpation: Only indirectly— behind the last molar, with the mouth opened half-way, between the maxillary tuber and lateral wing of the pterygoid process.

   Symptomatology: Indicator for the presence of parafunctions:

- Frontal bruxism
- Eccentric bruxism

Projected Pain:

- Pain more likely in deep location
- Into the ear
- Into the temporomandibular joint
- Into the tongue
- Into the floor of the mouth
- Into the maxillary sinus

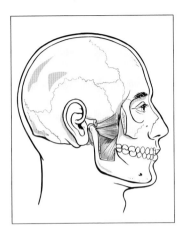

► **Fig. 42.4** Gnathologic aspects of the lateral pterygoid muscle.

43 Short Muscles of the Neck

Description of the Muscles

▶ Fig. 43.1

The posterior arch of the atlas is located in the suboccipital triangle, formed by the superior and inferior oblique muscles and the rectus capitis posterior major muscle. The vertebral artery runs on its superior border in a posteromedial direction, after passing through the transverse foramen and before entering the foramen magnum to merge with the basilar artery. In this region, injection and dry-needling pose an increased risk to the artery.

Origin:
- Rectus capitis posterior minor muscle: posterior tubercle of the atlas
- Rectus capitis posterior major muscle: spinous process of the axis
- Superior oblique muscle of the head: transverse process of the atlas
- Inferior oblique muscle of the head: spinous process of the axis

Insertion:
- Rectus capitis posterior minor muscle: medial portion of the inferior nuchal line of the occipital bone
- Rectus capitis posterior major muscle: lateral portion of the inferior nuchal line
- Superior oblique muscle of head: occipital bone, superior and lateral to the inferior nuchal line
- Inferior oblique muscle of the head: transverse process of the atlas

Innervation:
- Rectus capitis posterior minor muscle and superior oblique muscle of the head: posterior branch of the occipital nerve (dorsal ramus of spinal nerve C1)
- Rectus capitis posterior major muscle: posterior branches of the occipital nerve (dorsal rami of spinal nerves C1 and C2)
- Inferior oblique muscle of the head: occipital nerve C2

Action: The muscles act on the atlanto-occipital joint and, for biomechanical reasons, cause minor ipsilateral rotation and simultaneous contralateral inclination of the head. When acting on the atlanto-axial joint, they rotate the head to the ipsilateral side.

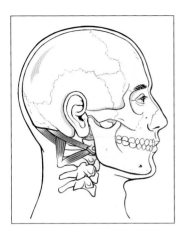

▶ **Fig. 43.1** Short neck muscles.

Trigger Points of the Short Neck Muscles

▶ Fig. 43.2

Introduction: Trigger points are frequently located in this region. They are caused more frequently by chronic rather than acute strain of the head joints. They predominantly develop when the vagus nerve is affected by increased visceral afferent signals. The close association of vertebral joints and the vagus nerve leads secondarily to poor posture, accompanied by trigger points. Headaches, vertigo, and acute strain are also conceivable in the context of whiplash injuries of the cervical spine. However, they more likely result from visceral afflictions of the left kidney, the parenchyma of which is innervated by the vagus nerve. People who regularly have to perform work above their head also tend to develop trigger points in this region as a result of muscle contraction.

Examination of trigger points: Detailed examination of the short neck muscles is normally not possible in a seated patient, because the overlaying muscles also usually exhibit increased tone. It is therefore advisable to palpate the short neck muscles with the patient in supine position. This kind of examination requires precise anatomical knowledge.

Trigger point therapy: Eliminating the cause of chronic poor posture is crucial. In most cases, it is necessary to first clear the visceral afferent signals osteopathically. Occipital release is highly recommended to relax the occipital muscles. In cases of severe muscle contraction, dry-needling and injection therapy are also an option. Follow-up treatment involves stretching of the short neck muscles by flexing the head joints and rotating the head to the contralateral side.

Trigger Points and Pain Projection Areas

Trigger points are located in the middle of the belly of the rectus capitis posterior major muscle and the inferior oblique muscle of the head. Pain is projected in an anterior direction across the occipital bone to the temporal bone. Maximum pain is felt in the region above the ear.

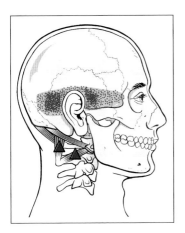

▶ **Fig. 43.2** Trigger points of the short neck muscles.

Important Acupuncture Points

▶ Fig. 43.3

GB-20

Location: In a depression between the insertions of the sternocleidomastoid muscle and trapezius muscle, at the lower edge of the occiput. The needle is inserted at the level between occiput and atlas (upper head joints) in the region of the transverse process of the atlas. It passes through the splenius muscle of the head then through the semispinalis muscle of the head and becomes positioned close to the superior and inferior oblique muscles of the head.

BL-10

Location: Above the first palpable spinous process of the cervical spine (C2, the axis), in the trapezius muscle where its belly just begins to descend. BL-10 is located about 0.5 Cun cranial to the dorsal hairline and lateral to GV-15, close to the exit of the greater occipital nerve.

Orientation on the horizontal axis is above the spinous process of C2 (axis).

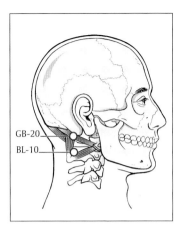

▶ **Fig. 43.3** GB-20 and BL-10.

44 Splenius Muscle of the Head

Description of the Muscle

▶ Fig. 44.1

Origin: Nuchal ligament at vertebrae C3 to C7 and spinous processes of vertebrae T1 and T2.

Insertion: Mastoid process of the temporal bone and superior nuchal line of the occipital bone, with slightly converging fibers running cranial and upward in lateral directions.

Innervation: Dorsal rami of the posterior branches of spinal nerves C3 to C5.

Action: Unilateral contraction of the muscle inclines the head and rotates it to the ipsilateral side. Bilateral contraction extends the head joints.

Trigger Points

Introduction: There is one trigger point near the insertion at the mastoid process. Trigger points in this region develop acutely as a result of wrong movements, for example, a failed forward summersault, or straining of soft neck tissues in connection with whiplash injury of the cervical spine.

On the other hand, increased tone of this muscle region is often associated with poor posture of the cervical spine caused by severe high thoracic kyphosis with reactive hyperextension of the cervical spine. In such cases, trigger points are also often observed in other muscles that extend the upper cervical spine, such as the short neck muscles.

Examination of trigger points: With the patient seated, palpate the trigger points directly in the region of the muscle insertions. A typical referred pain can often be induced.

Trigger point therapy: Treatment of the splenius muscle of the head is performed directly by dry-needling or infiltration of the trigger point. Extreme caution is advised for dry-needling or infiltration in the region of the two uppermost transverse processes because of the risk of damaging the vertebral artery and emerging nerves. The risk of injuring the vertebral artery and emerging nerves is minimized by needling from cranial to caudal while palpating the transverse process. Follow-up treatment involves stretching the

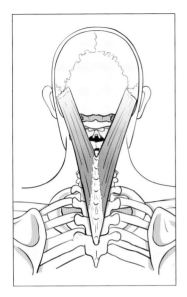

▶ **Fig. 44.1** Splenius muscle of the head.

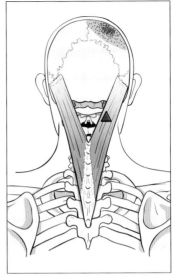

▶ **Fig. 44.2** Trigger points, splenius muscle of the head.

muscle by bending of the head laterally and rotating it to the contralateral side while flexing the cervical spine at the same time.

Trigger Points and Pain Projection Areas

Trigger point: Located near the tranverse processes of the upper two to three cervical vertebrae (▶ Fig. 44.2). The pain radiates predominantly into the ipsilateral occipital bone, rarely diffusely into the face or forehead.

Important Acupuncture Points

▶ Fig. 44.3

GB-20

Location: In a depression between the insertions of the sternocleidomastoid muscle and trapezius muscle at the lower edge of the occiput. The needle is inserted at the level between occiput and atlas (upper head joints) in the region of the transverse process of the atlas. It passes through the splenius muscle of the head then through the semispinalis muscle of the head and becomes positioned close to the superior and inferior oblique muscles of the head.

BL-10

Location: Above the first palpable spinous process of the cervical spine (C2, the axis), in the trapezius muscle where its belly just begins to descend. It is located about 0.5 Cun lateral to GV-15, close to the exit of the greater occipital nerve.

Orientation on the horizontal axis is above the spinous process of C2 (the axis).

GV-14

Location: Inferior to the spinous process of vertebra C7.

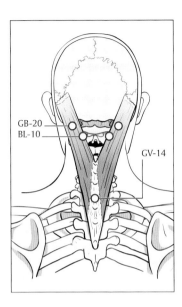

▶ **Fig. 44.3** GB-20, BL-10, and GV-14.

45 Anterior, Middle, and Posterior Scalene Muscles

Description of the Muscle

Anterior Scalene Muscle

▶ Fig. 45.1

Origin: Anterior tubercles of the transverse processes of vertebrae C3 to C6.

Insertion: Anterior scalene tubercle of the first rib.

Innervation: Anterior branches of spinal nerves C5 to C8.

Action: With the first rib fixed, it flexes the cervical spine to the ipsilateral side and rotates it to the contralateral side. With the cervical spine fixed, it raises the first rib and supports inspiration.

Middle Scalene Muscle

▶ Fig. 45.2

Origin: Anterior tubercles of the transverse processes of vertebrae C2 to C7.

Insertion: First rib, posterior to the subclavian sulcus and at the external intercostal membrane of the first intercostal space.

Innervation: Anterior branches of spinal nerves C4 to C8.

Action: Flexes the cervical spine laterally. With the cervical spine fixed, raises the first and second ribs. Auxiliary respiratory muscle supporting inspiration.

Posterior Scalene Muscle

▶ Fig. 45.3

Origin: Posterior tubercles of the transverse processes of vertebrae C5 and C6.

Insertion: Superior border of the second rib.

Innervation: Anterior branches of spinal nerves C6 to C8.

Action: Flexes the cervical spine laterally. With the cervical spine fixed, raises the first and second rib. Auxiliary respiratory muscle supporting inspiration.

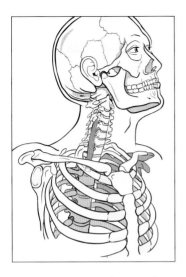

▶ **Fig. 45.1** Anterior scalene muscle.

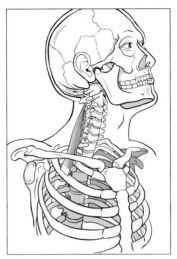

▶ **Fig. 45.2** Middle scalene muscle.

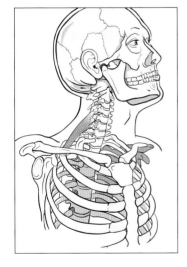

▶ **Fig. 45.3** Posterior scalene muscle.

ℹ Additional Information

The anterior scalene hiatus is formed by the posterior border of the clavicular part of the sternoclei-domastoid muscle and the anterior border of the anterior scalene muscle. This is where the subclavian vein is located. The subclavian artery and the brachial plexus pass through the posterior scalene hiatus between the posterior border of the anterior scalene muscle and the anterior border of the middle scalene muscle.

Trigger Points

Introduction: Acute causes for trigger points in this muscle group are distortion traumas of the cervical spine with primarily lateral impact. Other causes include sleeping in an unfavorable position. Chronic strain occurs particularly when the scalene muscles are used as auxiliary respiratory muscles, for example, with bronchial asthma.

Trigger points are frequently located in the middle scalene muscle, usually in association with trigger points in the superior trapezius, the sternocleidomastoid muscles, and the splenius muscle of the head. These trigger points are clinically relevant in the context of thoracic outlet and thoracic inlet syndromes. Thoracic outlet syndrome is caused by compression of the subclavian and vertebral arteries and the brachial plexus. Symptoms reported by patients are cold hands and paresthesia affecting the entire hand and forearm and occurring especially at night, but also when lifting or carrying heavy loads.

This compression syndrome is very common and is often confused with carpal tunnel syndrome. Electrophysiological studies have revealed a reduced velocity of nerve conduction. This not only affects the median nerve, but also the radial and ulnar nerves. On the other hand, compression of the subclavian vein and of lymphatic drainage in the anterior scalene hiatus causes swelling of the hand. This is quite often reported by patients and is known as thoracic inlet syndrome.

Examination of trigger points: Palpate trigger points in the anterior scalene muscle ventral and dorsal to the sternocleidomastoid muscle, and those of the posterior scalene muscle dorsal to the sternocleidomastoid muscle. The posterior scalene muscle is flatter than the middle scalene muscle and is partly covered by the levator muscle of the scapula. The insertion on the second rib is usually not palpable.

Trigger point therapy: Trigger points in the middle scalene muscle are well accessible to infiltration or dry-needling. Needling must not be too deep in order to avoid damage to the spinal nerves. One should keep in mind that the pleural cupula extends in a superior (cranial) direction beyond the clavicular level. Injection into the anterior and posterior scalene muscles should only be performed by a very experienced therapist. Particularly in the anterior portion, great care must be taken to ensure that the injection or acupuncture of the trigger point is performed laterally to the common carotid artery. Follow-up treatment involves lateral flexion of the cervical spine with fixed shoulder girdle.

Trigger Points and Pain Projection Areas

▶ Fig. 45.4, ▶ Fig. 45.5, ▶ Fig. 45.6

Trigger points: Precise delineation of individual trigger points is not required. The most accessible trigger point is located in the caudal portion of the middle scalene muscle. The pain radiates mainly into the medial border of the scapula, from the dorsal upper arm to the elbow and lateral to the biceps muscle. It also radiates into the forearm along the extensors of the first and second fingers and into the anterior portion of the brachioradial muscle, causing maximum pain in the dorsal sides of the index finger and thumb.

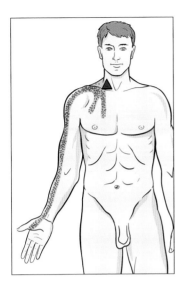

▶ **Fig. 45.4** Scalene muscles, trigger points (1).

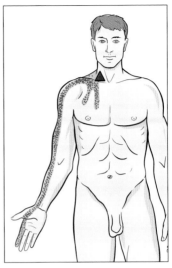

▶ **Fig. 45.5** Scalene muscles, trigger points (2).

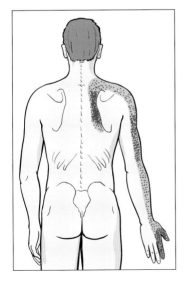

▶ **Fig. 45.6** Scalene muscles, trigger points (3).

Important Acupuncture Points

▶ Fig. 45.7, ▶ Fig. 45.8, ▶ Fig. 45.9

SI-16

Location: At the posterior border of the sternocleidomastoid muscle, at the level of the laryngeal prominence.

SI-17

Location: Inferior to the earlobe, in front of the sternocleidomastoid muscle, at the level of the inferior border of the mandible.

ST-9

Location: At the level of the thyroid cartilage, just in front of the sternocleidomastoid muscle. The pulsation of the carotid artery is palpable here.

ST-10

Location: Anterior border of the sternocleidomastoid muscle, in the middle of the line connecting ST-9 to ST-11.

ST-11

Location: On the upper border of the clavicle, between the sternal clavicular insertions of the sternocleidomastoid muscle, at the transition between the shaft and the medial head of the clavicle (superior to point KI-27.)

ST-12

Location: In the supraclavicular fossa, 4 Cun lateral to the median line, lateral to the clavicular part of the sternocleidomastoid muscle.

ST-13

Location: On the lower border of the clavicle, 4 Cun lateral to the anterior median line.

ST-14

Location: In the first intercostal space (ICS), on the mammillary line, 4 Cun lateral to the anterior median line.

ST-17

Location: In the ICS, 4 Cun lateral to the anterior median line.

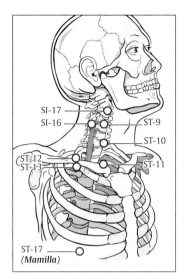

▶ **Fig. 45.7** SI-16, SI-17, ST-9, and ST-10.

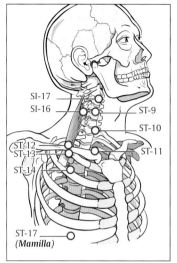

▶ **Fig. 45.8** ST-11, ST-12, and ST-13.

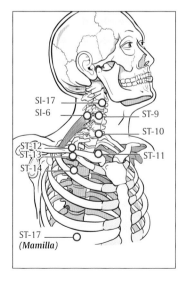

▶ **Fig. 45.9** ST-14 and ST-17.

46 Trapezius Muscle

▶ Fig. 46.1, ▶ Fig. 46.2

Description of the Muscle

Origin:
- Descending part: the outer occipital protuberance to cervical vertebra C6
- Transverse part: from spinous process of C7 to spinous process of thoracic vertebra T3
- Ascending part: vertebrae T3 to T12

Insertion: Lateral third of clavicle, acromion and spine of the scapula.

Innervation: Accessory nerve (11th cranial nerve).

Action: The muscle performs a broad range of movements in the shoulder region. Among others, it elevates the shoulder (ascending and descending part), retracts the scapula medially (transverse part), and moves the head when the shoulder girdle is fixed (dorsal extension when contracted on both sides).

Trigger Points of the Trapezius Muscle

▶ Fig. 46.3, ▶ Fig. 46.4

Introduction: The trapezius muscle encompasses seven trigger point areas. Activation of these trigger points results predominantly from chronic strain as a result of poor posture, constant sitting, scoliosis, as well as physically unbalanced occupational activities (e.g., typing). Less often it results from acute traumas. Trigger points in this muscle are especially common in cases of psychogenic stress. These trigger points are associated with points in the levator muscle of the scapula or in the scalene muscles as well as in the sternocleidomastoid muscle and pectoral muscles.

Examination of trigger points: Palpate these points either by using the thumb or by a pinch grip with thumb and index finger. In addition to triggered pain projections, shortened muscle structures where violent local twitch responses can be triggered are frequently a characteristic feature. Examination is usually performed with the patient seated, with a rounded back and simultaneously grasping the opposite upper arm with the hand.

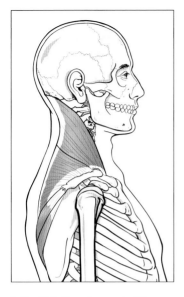

▶ **Fig. 46.1** Trapezius muscle (1).

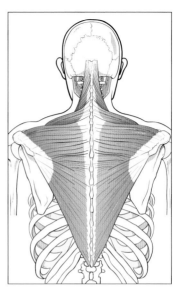

▶ **Fig. 46.2** Trapezius muscle (2).

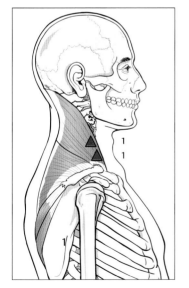

▶ **Fig. 46.3** Trigger points of the trapezius muscle (1).

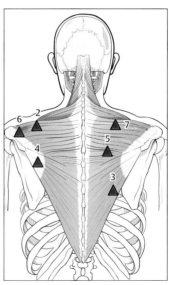

▶ **Fig. 46.4** Trigger points of the trapezius muscle (2).

Trigger point therapy: Conventional acupuncture. Therapeutic local anesthesia and intramuscular stimulation to loosen up the taut bands. Follow-up treatment by means of passive stretching of the muscular structures.

Trigger Points and Pain Projection Areas

Trigger point 1: Located at the anterior margin of the clavicular part (▶ **Fig. 46.5**) and typically radiates toward the mastoid, mandibular angle, and into the area above the lateral eyebrow. Inconstant pain projections between the tip of the mastoid process and the ascending part of the lower jaw and also within a semicircular strip from the mastoid process via the occipital bone and temporal bone up to the temporal region.

Trigger point 2: Located in the transverse part at the transition from the medial third to the lateral third (▶ **Fig. 46.6**). Its main pain projection area is dorsomedial to the mastoid process and also extends in a weaker form from the trigger point to the main projection area.

Trigger point 3: Located 2 Cun medial to the medial margin of the scapula at the level of the spinous process of T6 (▶ **Fig. 46.6**).

Its main pain projection area extends into the region of the acromial and nuchal insertions of the muscle. A secondary projection area is the entire area of the muscle above the trigger point.

Trigger point 4: Located 1 to 2 Cun lateral to the medial margin in a depression below the scapular spine (▶ **Fig. 46.7**). Its main pain projection area is at the medial margin of the scapula.

Trigger point 5: Located just medial to the medial scapular margin, approximately 2 Cun above the scapular spine (▶ **Fig. 46.7**). The pain projection area is localized between C6 and T3, immediately adjacent to the vertebrae, and extends in a weakened form into the transverse part of the trapezius muscle.

Trigger point 6: Located close to the insertion at the dorsal acromion (▶ **Fig. 46.7**), which is also its area of pain projection.

Trigger point 7: Located in a region approximately 5 × 5 cm in the middle of the transverse part of the trapezius muscle (▶ **Fig. 46.8**). Projects pain along the lateral upper arm and into the lateral epicondyle of the humerus.

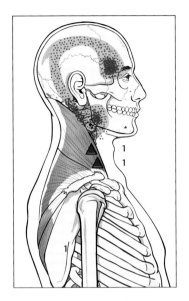

▶ **Fig. 46.5** Trapezius muscle, trigger point 1.

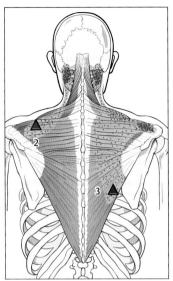

▶ **Fig. 46.6** Trapezius muscle, trigger points 2 and 3.

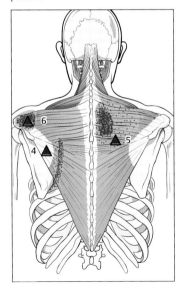

▶ **Fig. 46.7** Trapezius muscle, trigger points 4, 5, and 6.

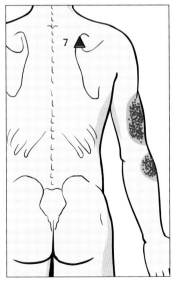

▶ **Fig. 46.8** Trapezius muscle, trigger point 7.

Important Acupuncture Points

▶ Fig. 46.9, ▶ Fig. 46.10

BL-10

Location:
- Vertical axis orientation: 1.3 Cun lateral to the posterior median line (Governing Vessel) in the muscle belly of the trapezius muscle (where it just begins to descend). BL-10 is lateral to GV-15, close to the exit of the greater occipital nerve
- Horizontal orientation: above the spinous process of C2 (axis)

BL-11

Location: 1.5 Cun lateral to the lower edge of the spinous process of T1.

BL-12

Location: 1.5 Cun lateral to the lower edge of the spinous process of T2.

GB-20

Location: In a depression between the insertions of the sternocleidomastoid muscle and trapezius muscle, in the region of the external occipital protuberance.

GV-14

Location: Below the spinous process of C7.

GV-15

Location: Above the spinous process of C2, at the same level as BL-10; 0.5 Cun above the dorsal hairline.

GV-16

Location: Below the external occipital protuberance, at the same level as GB-20.

BL-13

Location: 1.5 Cun lateral to the lower edge of the spinous process of T3.

BL-14

Location: 1.5 Cun lateral to the lower edge of the spinous process of T4.

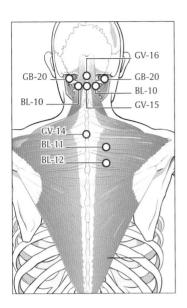

▶ **Fig. 46.9** BL-10, 11, and 12, GB-20, GV-14, 15, and 16.

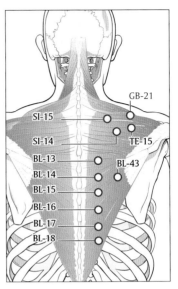

▶ **Fig. 46.10** BL-13, 14, 15, 16, 17, 18, and 43, SE-14, TE-15, and GB-21.

BL-15

Location: 1.5 Cun lateral to the lower edge of the spinous process of T5.

BL-16

Location: 1.5 Cun lateral to the lower edge of the spinous process of T6.

BL-17

Location: 1.5 Cun lateral to the lower edge of the spinous process of T7.

BL-18

Location: 1.5 Cun lateral to the lower edge of the spinous process of T9.

BL-43

Location: 3 Cun lateral to the median line, below the lower edge of the spinous process of T4.

SI-14

Location: 3 Cun lateral to the spinous process of T1.

SI-15

Location: 2 Cun lateral to the lower edge of the spinous process of C7.

TE-15

Location: Midway between GB-21 and SI-13, over the superior angle of the scapula. TE-15 is located approximately 1 Cun caudal to GB-21.

GB-21

Location: In the center of the connecting line between the acromion and spinous process of C7, on the dorsal elongation of a line through the mammillary.

Gnathologic Aspects

Trapezius Muscle, Transverse Part

▶ Fig. 46.11, ▶ Fig. 46.12
Functional aspects:
- Bilateral activity: extends the cervical spine and thoracic spine
- Unilateral activity: raises, rotates, and retracts the scapula
- Mediotrusion in a narrower sense: masticatory muscle; stabilizes the neck during chewing

Palpation: Upper margin: from neck to acromion.
Symptomatology:
- Occipital headache
- Shoulder pain
- Stiff shoulder
- Increases all pain in the masticatory muscles, especially in the temporal muscle, masseter muscle, lateral pterygoid muscle, and sternocleidomastoid muscle

Projected pain:
- Into the neck
- Occipital, in the insertion area of the splenius muscle of the head
- Extends from behind the ear, across the ear and into the temporal region
- Into the submaxillary angle
- Into molars of the lower jaw
- Vertigo

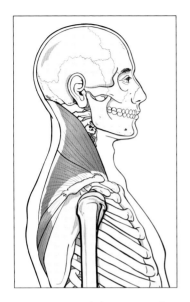

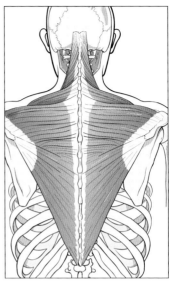

▶ **Fig. 46.11** Gnathologic aspects of the trapezius muscle, transverse part (1).

▶ **Fig. 46.12** Gnathologic aspects of the trapezius muscle, transverse part (2).

47 Levator Muscle of the Scapula

Description of the Muscle

▶ Fig. 47.1

Origin: Posterior tubercles of transverse processes of C1 to C4.
Insertion: Superior angle of the scapula.
Innervation: Dorsal nerve of the scapula (C3 to C5).
Action: Retracts scapula after elevation.

Trigger Points

Introduction: The two trigger points of the levator muscle of the scapula frequently cause ongoing severe discomfort. They can be activated by acute strain (e.g., long car drives) but primarily by chronic contraction of the muscles through increased innervation of the postural muscles due to poor posture. Less often, these trigger points are activated in tennis players and in swimmers, or in connection with infections. Activation is also observed with constant use of forearm crutches and with psychosomatic disorders.

Examination of trigger points: Patients are examined while lying on their side, with the head supported in order to avoid lateral flexion of the cervical spine. The trigger points are palpated directly on the insertion at the superior angle of the scapula and in the part of the muscle above the superior angle of the scapula, respectively. Typically, pronounced taut bands are palpated close to the insertion.

Trigger point therapy: Conventional acupuncture to deactivate trigger points. Intramuscular stimulation or trigger point infiltration to release taut bands. Active stretching of the muscle is performed on the seated patient by fixing the ipsilateral shoulder (e.g., on a chair) and passive stretching through inclination and lateral flexion of the cervical spine using postisometric relaxation.

Trigger Points and Pain Projection Areas

Trigger points 1 and 2: Trigger point 1 is located close to the medial margin of the superior angle of the scapula. Trigger point

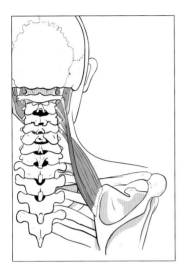

▶ **Fig. 47.1** Levator muscle of the scapula.

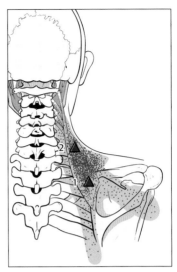

▶ **Fig. 47.2** Levator muscle of the scapula, trigger points 1 and 2.

2 is located at the transition between the transverse part and descending part of the trapezius muscle (▶ **Fig. 47.2**). Pain projection areas surround the trigger points and radiate into the upper dorsolateral part of the deltoid muscle and along the medial margin of the scapula.

Important Acupuncture Points

▶ Fig. 47.3

SI-14

Location: 3 Cun lateral to the spinous process of T1.

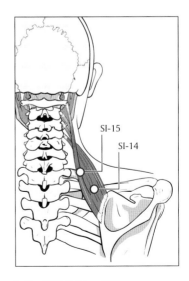

▶ **Fig. 47.3** SI-14 and 15.

SI-15

Location: 2 Cun lateral to the lower edge of the spinous process of C7.

Gnathologic Aspects

▶ Fig. 47.4

Functional aspects:
- Elevates scapula
- Rotates the neck when the scapula is fixed
- Responsible for symmetry of head posture
- Helps with lifting and carrying heavy loads
- Masticatory muscle in narrower sense because it stabilizes head posture while chewing
- Often painful in case of parafunction

Palpation: Medial to the cranial angle of the clavicle.

> **Caution!**
> Can be confused with the upper margin of the trapezius muscle.

Symptomatology:
- Torticollis
- Shoulder pain at the transition to the neck
- Driver's neck pain
- Stiff neck
- Stiff shoulder

Projected pain:
- Lateral into the neck
- Into the superior angle of the scapula

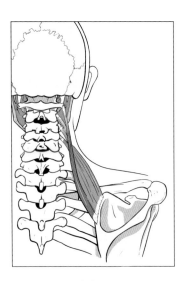

▶ **Fig. 47.4** Gnathologic aspect of the levator muscle of the scapula.

48   Sternocleidomastoid Muscle

Description of the Muscle

▶ Fig. 48.1

Origin:
- Sternal head: upper margin of the manubrium of the sternum
- Clavicular head: upper margin of the medial third of the clavicle

Insertion: Mastoid process and extending toward the superior nuchal line of the occipital bone.

Innervation: Accessory nerve (11th cranial nerve).

Action:
- Unilateral contraction: ipsilateral flexion and rotation to the opposite side
- Bilateral contraction: dorsal extension of the cervical spine

Note: The main branches of the cervical plexus arise from the middle third of the muscle's posterior margin. The carotid triangle, with the ramification of the common carotid artery and the first branches of the external carotid artery, is located at about the same level of the muscle's anterior margin.

Trigger Points

Introduction: There are seven trigger points (▶ Fig. 48.2): four in the sternal portion of the sternocleidomastoid muscle and three in the clavicular portion. Activating factors include: chronic muscle strain, especially due to scoliosis, but also sternosymphyseal strain posture; chronic strain or reactions, for example, after cervical whiplash injury or hangover headache after excessive alcohol consumption; chronic sinusitis or tooth infection. Rare causes are leakage after cerebrospinal fluid puncture or nucleotomy. Associated trigger points are mainly localized in the contralateral sternocleidomastoid muscle, but also in all dorsal neck muscles and in the temporomandibular system. In the area of the lower trigger points of the sternal portion, arthritis of the sternoclavicular joint should be ruled out by differential diagnosis. Differential diagnosis should also consider ear, nose, and throat disorders such as Ménière's disease, Horton's syndrome (cluster headache), and torticollis in the broadest sense.

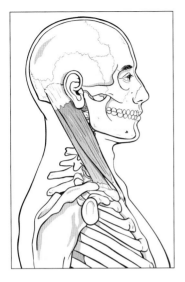

▶ **Fig. 48.1** Sternocleidomastoid muscle.

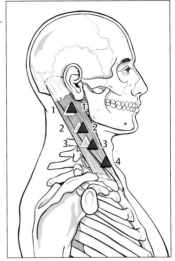

▶ **Fig. 48.2** Trigger points of the sternocleidomastoid muscle.

Examination of trigger points:
With the patient seated and the head fixed in neutral position, use a pinch grip to thoroughly palpate the sternal portion of the sternocleidomastoid muscle. The deeper portions of the clavicular part are best examined using a pinch grip while the patient is lying down and the cervical spine is flexed ipsilaterally. Again, one should distinguish between taut bands and pain projection areas.

Trigger point therapy: Conventional needling of trigger points; if indicated, inactivation by means of therapeutic local anesthesia and release of taut bands by means of intramuscular stimulation while avoiding the underlying vascular and neural structures. Passive stretching of the clavicular part through rotation of the head toward the opposite side, moderate reclination and simultaneous lateral flexion to the opposite side. Stretching of the sternal part is achieved through ipsilateral rotation with ipsilateral flexion. Postisometric relaxation can also be helpful.

Trigger Points and Pain Projection Areas

Trigger points 1 to 4 (sternal part): The pain projection areas for the four trigger points of the sternal part of the sternocleidomastoid muscle are in the occipital region above the mastoid process and at the level of the sternoclavicular joint. An arched area of projected pain starts at the medial side of the eyebrow and radiates laterally toward the ear and the zygomatic arch (▶ **Fig. 48.3**). Inconstant areas of pain are described at the level of upper and lower jaw, tip of the chin, below the mandible and in the region of the parietal bone.

Trigger points 1 to 3 (clavicular part): The pain projection areas for the three trigger points of the clavicular part are primarily at the level of the ear, behind the auricula, and in the front above both eyes (▶ **Fig. 48.4**).

Important Acupuncture Points

▶ Fig. 48.5, ▶ Fig. 48.6

LI-17

Location: 1 Cun caudal to LI-18, at the posterior margin of the sternocleidomastoid muscle.

LI-18

Location: At the level of the thyroid cartilage, between the sternal and clavicular heads of the sternocleidomastoid muscle.

SI-16

Location: Posterior margin of the sternocleidomastoid muscle, at the level of the laryngeal prominence.

TE-17

Location: Behind the ear lobe, between the lower jaw and mastoid process.

ST-9

Location: At the level of the thyroid cartilage, immediately in front of the sternocleidomastoid muscle. Pulsation of the carotid artery is palpable here.

ST-10

Location: Anterior margin of the sternocleidomastoid muscle, in the middle of the connecting line between ST-9 and ST-11. (Note: ST-11 is below ST-9, at the upper margin of the clavicle, between the two heads of the sternocleidomastoid muscle.)

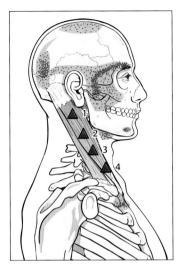

▶ **Fig. 48.3** Sternocleidomastoid muscle, trigger points 1 to 4 (sternal portion).

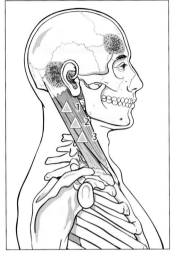

▶ **Fig. 48.4** Sternocleidomastoid muscle, trigger points 1 to 3 (clavicular portion).

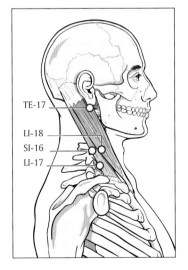

▶ **Fig. 48.5** SI-16, LI-17, LI-18, and TE-17.

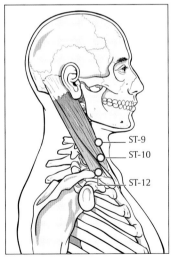

▶ **Fig. 48.6** ST-9, 10, and 12.

ST-12

Location: Center of the supraclavicular fossa, 4 Cun lateral to the median line as well as lateral to the clavicular part of the sternocleidomastoid muscle.

Gnathologic Aspects

▶ Fig. 48.7

Functional aspects:
- Bilateral activity: holds head in upright position
- Unilateral activity: "dove posture," that is
  - rotates the head to the opposite side
  - inclines the head on the same side
  - raises the chin (the head) on the opposite side

Palpation:
- Insertion at the mastoid process
- Sternal origin
- Clavicular origin
- At various positions in the muscle's belly

Symptomatology: Poor posture of the head toward the front, headache of any localization (called "atypical" facial neuralgia, tension headache, and cervical cephalgia), hemicrania.

Projected pain:
- No neck pain
- Sternal portion:
  - into the crown of the head
  - into the occiput
  - into the eye, around the eye and deep behind the eye (often with increased lacrimation, reddened conjunctiva, ptosis [drooping of the upper eyelid], vision problems)
  - two-dimensionally into the lateral face (often erroneously called "atypical facial pain")
  - across the cheek
  - into the lateral upper jaw
  - into the acoustic meatus
  - into the region of the hyoid bone and larynx
  - difficulty in swallowing and sensation of sore throat
  - into the sternum
  - into a small spot lateral to the chin
  - sometimes ringing in the ears or even tinnitus
- Clavicular portion:
  - toward the front: frontal headache
  - in the front, often also from the ipsilateral direction
  - projecting in a contralateral direction and into the ear (often confused with otitis media)

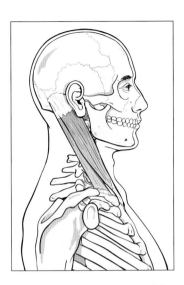

▶ **Fig. 48.7** Gnathologic aspects of the sternocleidomastoid muscle.

- Retroauricular portion:
  - into the cheek
  - diffuse into the teeth of the lateral upper jaw
  - dizziness, with perceived movements and sensations in the head, rarely vertigo
  - disequilibrium

49 Subclavius Muscle

Description of the Muscle

▶ Fig. 49.1

Origin: Cranial surface of the first rib, near the bone–cartilage junction.

Insertion: Lower surface of clavicle.

Innervation: Subclavian nerve (C5 to C6).

Action: Lowers the acromial end of the clavicle and presses it against the sternum. This muscle also forms a cushion between the first rib and the clavicle and maintains the flow of blood and lymph in the subclavicular vessels, particularly in the subclavian vein and lymph vessels. This function counteracts a thoracic inlet syndrome.

Trigger Points

Introduction: Trigger points often develop here as a result of thoracic inlet syndrome. Trigger points in this region are frequently found in association with trigger points of the smaller and greater pectoral muscles.

Examination of trigger points: This muscle is best palpated using a pinch grip, with patients in the lateral position. Painful myogelosis is often found beneath the lateral part of the clavicle.

Trigger point therapy: The most successful treatment is acupressure, which can be combined with simultaneous mobilization of the shoulder girdle. The patient is in a lateral position with the affected side facing upward. The therapist stands behind the patient and grasps the clavicle with one hand, while the other hand touches the back of the shoulder girdle and performs rotations by moving the shoulder girdle in cranial, ventral, caudal, and dorsal directions.

> ┌─ Caution! ─────────────
> Acupuncture or injection of these trigger points poses a risk of damaging the pleura.

Trigger Points and Pain Projection Areas

Trigger point 1: Pain usually occurs in the clavicular area itself; it also radiates into the anterior upper arm and into the radial side of the dorsal and ventral forearm (▶ Fig. 49.2, ▶ Fig. 49.3).

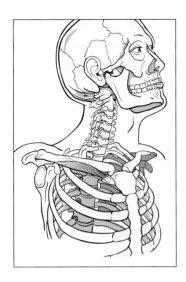

▶ **Fig. 49.1** Subclavius muscle.

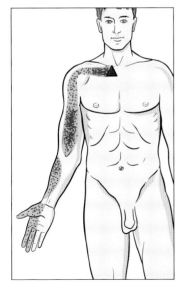

▶ **Fig. 49.2** Subclavius muscle, trigger point 1 (1).

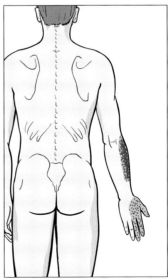

▶ **Fig. 49.3** Subclavius muscle, trigger point 1 (2).

Important Acupuncture Points

▶ Fig. 49.4

LU-1

Location: 6 Cun lateral to the median line, 1 Cun below the clavicle, slightly medial to the caudal border of the coracoid process, at the level of the first intercostal space (ICS 1).

LU-2

Location: Directly below the clavicle, at about the same distance from the median line as LU-1.

ST-11

Location: On the upper border of the clavicle, between the sternal clavicular insertions of the sternocleidomastoid muscle, at the transition between the shaft and the medial head of the clavicle (superior to KI-27).

ST-12

Location: In the middle of the supraclavicular fossa, 4 Cun lateral to the median line, lateral to the clavicular part of the sternocleidomastoid muscle.

ST-13

Location: On the lower border of the clavicle, 4 Cun lateral to the anterior median line.

KI-27

Location: Just below the clavicle, 2 Cun lateral to the anterior median line and close to the sternoclavicular joint.

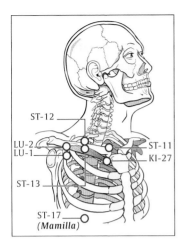

▶ **Fig. 49.4** LU-1, 2, ST-11, 12, 13, and KI-27.

50 Greater Pectoral Muscle

Description of the Muscle

▶ Fig. 50.1

Origin:
- Clavicular part: medial half of the clavicle
- Sternocostal part: anterior plane of the sternum and costal cartilages of the six upper ribs
- Abdominal part: anterior plate of the rectus sheath

Insertion: Crest of the lesser tubercle of the humerus (lower parts insert most cranially).

Innervation: Medial and lateral pectoral nerves (C5–T1).

Action: Adduction and inward rotation of the arm, retraction from elevation, accessory respiratory muscle.

Trigger Points

Introduction: This muscle has trigger points in five different areas according to its anatomical structure. Active trigger points can be expected with sterno-symphyseal strain posture, with shoulders rotated to the front; also with acute strain from carrying heavy items or in case of unaccustomed physical stress. However, symptoms with projection to the upper anterior thoracic region also appear in cases of symptomatic coronary heart disease and cardiac infarction ("heart attack"). Persistent symptoms following such an event point to active trigger points of the greater pectoral muscle.

Examination of trigger points: Direct palpation or using the pinch grip at the lateral part of the muscle can frequently trigger local twitch responses, if the muscle is stretched in a targeted manner by horizontal abduction of the arm and simultaneous retraction of the shoulder joints.

Trigger point therapy: Conventional needling or, alternatively, therapeutic local anesthesia and targeted release of taut bands using intramuscular stimulation. This is followed by passive stretching of the muscle, with the arm rotated outward and the shoulders retracted.

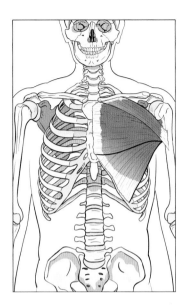

▶ **Fig. 50.1** Greater pectoral muscle.

Trigger Points and Pain Projection Areas

Trigger points 1 and 2 (clavicular part of the left greater pectoral muscle): There are two trigger points in the middle third of the clavicular head (▶ Fig. 50.2). Their main areas of projection are at the ventral portion of the deltoid muscle. This applies only to the left greater pectoral muscle.

Trigger points 3 to 5 (sternocostal part of the left greater pectoral muscle): The three trigger points of the sternocostal part (▶ Fig. 50.3) have their main projection areas directly over the greater pectoral muscle. Another projection area is located close to the origin, at the level of the ulnar flexor muscle of the wrist and on the inside of the upper arm as well as close to the middle and ring fingers. This applies only to the left greater pectoral muscle.

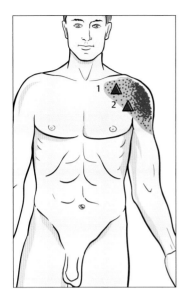

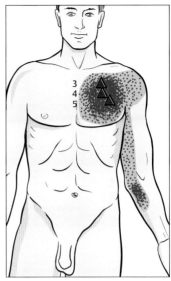

▶ **Fig. 50.2** Greater pectoral muscle (clavicular part, left greater pectoral muscle), trigger points 1 and 2.

▶ **Fig. 50.3** Greater pectoral muscle (sternocostal part, left greater pectoral muscle), trigger points 3 to 5.

Trigger points 1 and 2 (sterno-costal part of the right greater pectoral muscle): These two trigger points (▶ Fig. 50.4) are located close to the sternum in the sternocostal part of the greater pectoral muscle. They have their main pain projection areas in this region. This applies only to the right greater pectoral muscle.

Trigger point 3 (abdominal part of the right greater pectoral muscle): This trigger point (▶ Fig. 50.4) is located in the middle of the abdominal part of the muscle and shows a correlation with arrhythmic heartbeat. This applies only to the right greater pectoral muscle.

Trigger points 6 and 7 (abdominal part of the left greater pectoral muscle): The two trigger points of the abdominal part are located immediately in front of the muscle's entrance into the axillary fossa (▶ Fig. 50.5). Their main projection area is medial and distant to the trigger points, at the level of the mammilla. This applies only to the left greater pectoral muscle.

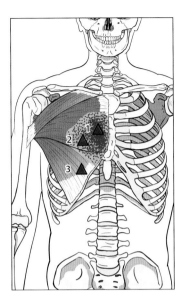

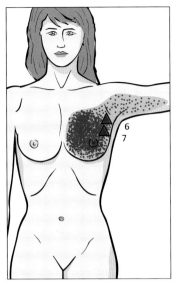

▶ **Fig. 50.4** Greater pectoral muscle (sternocostal part, right greater pectoral muscle), trigger points 1 and 2; greater pectoral muscle (abdominal part, right greater pectoral muscle), trigger point 3.

▶ **Fig. 50.5** Greater pectoral muscle (abdominal part, left greater pectoral muscle), trigger point 6 and 7.

Important Acupuncture Points

▶ Fig. 50.6, ▶ Fig. 50.7, ▶ Fig. 50.8

LU-1

Location: 6 Cun lateral to the anterior median line, 1 Cun below the clavicle, slightly medial to the caudal border of the coracoid process, at the level of the first intercostal space (ICS 1).

ST-13

Location: At the lower edge of the clavicle, 4 Cun lateral to the anterior median line.

ST-14

Location: Within ICS 1 on the mammillary line, 4 Cun lateral to the anterior median line.

ST-15

Location: Within ICS 2 on the mammillary line, 4 Cun lateral to the anterior median line.

ST-16

Location: Within ICS 3 on the mammillary line, 4 Cun lateral to the anterior median line.

ST-17

Location: Within ICS 4 at the mammilla, 4 Cun lateral to the anterior median line.

ST-18

Location: Within ICS 5 on the mammillary line, 4 Cun lateral to the anterior median line.

SP-18

Location: Within ICS 4, 2 Cun lateral and slightly cranial to the mammilla. (Note: the ascending aspect of the intercostal space.)

SP-19

Location: Within ICS 3, 2 Cun lateral to the mammillary line.

SP-20

Location: Within ICS 2, 2 Cun lateral to the cranially extended mammillary line.

KI-22

Location: Within ICS 5, 2 Cun lateral to the anterior median line.

KI-23

Location: Within ICS 4, 2 Cun lateral to the anterior median line.

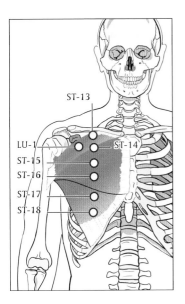

▶ **Fig. 50.6** LU-1, ST-13, 14, 15, 16, 17, and 18.

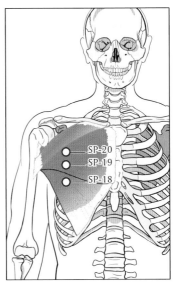

▶ **Fig. 50.7** SP-18, 19 and 20.

KI-24

Location: Within ICS 3, 2 Cun lateral to the anterior median line.

KI-25

Location: Within ICS 2, 2 Cun lateral to the anterior median line.

KI-26

Location: Within ICS 1, 2 Cun lateral to the anterior median line.

KI-27

Location: Directly under the clavicle, 2 Cun lateral to the anterior median line.

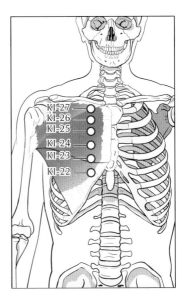

▶ **Fig. 50.8** KI-22, 23, 24, 25, 26 and 27.

51 Smaller Pectoral Muscle

Description of the Muscle

▶ Fig. 51.1

Origin: End of bony portions of the third to fifth ribs.
Insertion: Coracoid process of the scapula with a short, flat tendon (together with tendon of the coracobrachial muscle and short head of the biceps muscle of the arm).
Innervation: Medial (C8/T1) and lateral (C5–C7) pectoral nerves.
Action: Lowers the scapula; raises the ribs when the arm is fixed (accessory respiratory muscle).

Trigger Points of the Smaller Pectoral Muscle

Introduction: This muscle tends toward contraction. Clinically, due to physiological density in this area, neurovascular problems (thoracic outlet syndrome) are very evident, especially when the arm is rotated outward and abducted more than 140°, causing compression of the brachial artery and brachial nerve trunks. Two trigger point locations are known; however, they often appear in combination with trigger points of the greater pectoral muscle and subclavius muscle.

Examination of trigger points: These trigger points can be palpated directly in patients lying on their back, with their arm abducted approximately 80° and rotated outward. The trigger point close to the origin at the level of the fourth rib is palpated under the greater pectoral muscle with either the index finger or thumb after gripping the greater pectoral muscle using the pinch grip.

Trigger point therapy: With patients in the same examination position as described above, these trigger points can either be needled directly or inactivated by dry-needling or therapeutic local anesthesia. When treating the trigger point close to the insertion of the muscle, one should

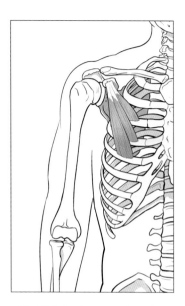

▶ **Fig. 51.1** Smaller pectoral muscle.

consider the risk of damaging the neurovascular structures underlying the tendon. Passive stretching of the muscle through abduction, external rotation, and retroversion of the arm using postisometric relaxation completes the treatment.

Trigger Points and Pain Projection Areas

Trigger points 1 and 2: There is only one area of pain projection for both trigger points (▶ Fig. 51.2). It is predominantly located over the anterior portion of the shoulder joint. The pain radiates across the thoracic muscles and along the entire ulnar side of the upper and lower arm and projects into the middle to little fingers. Trigger point 1 is located close to the insertion, approximately 1 to 2 Cun caudal to the coracoid process. Trigger point 2 is located close to the origin, at the level of the fourth rib.

Important Acupuncture Points

▶ Fig. 51.3

LU-1

Location: At the level of the first intercostal space (ICS 1), 6 Cun lateral to the anterior median line, 1 Cun below the clavicle, slightly medial to the caudal border of the coracoid process.

ST-15

Location: Within ICS 2 on the mammillary line, 4 Cun lateral to the anterior median line.

ST-16

Location: Within ICS 3 on the mammillary line, 4 Cun lateral to the anterior median line.

ST-17

Location: Within ICS 4 at the mammilla, 4 Cun lateral to the anterior median line.

SP-19

Location: Within ICS 3, 2 Cun lateral to the mammillary line.

SP-20

Location: Within ICS 2, 2 Cun lateral to the cranially extended mammillary line.

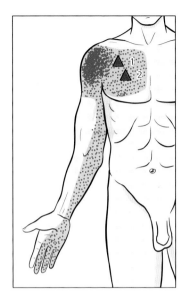

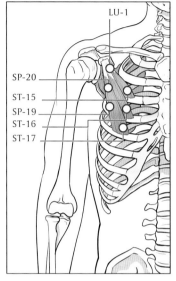

▶ **Fig. 51.2** Smaller pectoral muscle, trigger points 1 and 2.

▶ **Fig. 51.3** LU-1, ST-15, 16, 17, SP-19 and 20.

52 Smaller and Greater Rhomboid Muscles

Description of the Muscles

Smaller Rhomboid Muscle

▶ Fig. 52.1

Origin: Spinous processes of C6 and C7.
Insertion: Upper medial margin of the scapula.
Innervation: Dorsal nerve of the scapula (C4/5).
Action: Retraction of elevation.

Greater Rhomboid Muscle

▶ Fig. 52.1

Origin: Spinous processes of T1 to T4.
Insertion: Medial margin of the scapula.
Innervation: Dorsal nerve of the scapula (C4/5).
Action: Retraction from elevation.

Trigger Points

Introduction: There are two trigger points in the greater rhomboid muscle and one trigger point in the smaller rhomboid muscle (▶ Fig. 52.2). These trigger points are primarily activated by strain, especially by sternosymphyseal strain positions with rounded back. Associated trigger points can be located in the levator muscle of the scapula, the infraspinatus muscle, and the middle portion of the trapezius muscle.

Examination of trigger points: These trigger points can be easily identified at the medial margin of the scapula with the patient seated in a rounded-back position.

Trigger point therapy: These trigger points can be rapidly inactivated by means of dry-needling, conventional acupuncture, or therapeutic local anesthesia using the tangential puncture technique to avoid pneumothorax.

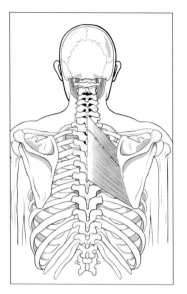

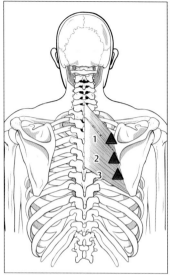

▶ **Fig. 52.1** Smaller and greater rhomboid muscles.

▶ **Fig. 52.2** Trigger points of the smaller and greater rhomboid muscles.

Trigger Points and Pain Projection Areas

Trigger points 1 to 3: The trigger point in the smaller rhomboid muscle is approximately 3 cm medial to the medial margin of the scapula. The two trigger points of the greater rhomboid muscle are located more caudally, again about 3 cm medial to the medial margin of the scapula. The pain projection areas for all three trigger points are located around the medial margin of the scapula and the supraspinous fossa (▶ **Fig. 52.3**).

Important Acupuncture Points

▶ Fig. 52.4

SI-14

Location: 3 Cun lateral to the lower edge of the spinous process of T1.

BL-11

Location: 1.5 Cun lateral to the lower edge of the spinous process of T1.

BL-12

Location: 1.5 Cun lateral to the lower edge of the spinous process of T2.

BL-13

Location: 1.5 Cun lateral to the lower edge of the spinous process of T3.

BL-14

Location: 1.5 Cun lateral to the lower edge of the spinous process of T4.

BL-41

Location: 3 Cun lateral to the lower edge of the spinous process of T2.

BL-42

Location: 3 Cun lateral to the lower edge of the spinous process of T3.

BL-43

Location: 3 Cun lateral to the lower edge of the spinous process of T4.

BL-44

Location: 3 Cun lateral to the lower edge of the spinous process of T5.

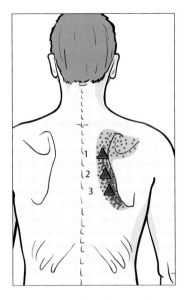

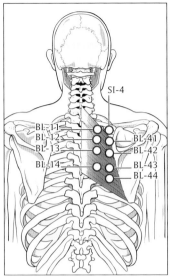

▶ **Fig. 52.3** Smaller and greater rhomboid muscles, trigger points 1 to 3.

▶ **Fig. 52.4** SI-14, BL-11, 12, 13, 14, 41, 42, 43, and 44.

53 Supraspinatus Muscle

Description of the Muscle

▶ Fig. 53.1

Origin: Supraspinous fossa of the scapula.

Insertion: Upper edge of the greater tubercle of the humerus, extending into the joint capsule (muscle of rotator cuff).

Innervation: Suprascapular nerve (C4–C6).

Action: Abduction; tightens the joint capsule.

Trigger Points

Introduction: There are three trigger points in this area, two of them in the muscle belly and one in the region of the supraspinous tendon (▶ Fig. 53.2). These trigger points are activated mostly in situations of acute strain (e.g., unaccustomed carrying of heavy loads), but also by chronic over-loading syndromes. These trigger points are usually associated with trigger points in the trapezius muscle, infraspinatus muscle, and latissimus dorsi muscle.

Examination of trigger points: These trigger points are directly palpated in the area of the muscle belly and close to the insertion, with the patient seated. Palpations trigger a typical referred pain.

Trigger point therapy: These trigger points are usually inactivated without any problem by acupuncture, therapeutic local anesthesia, or dry-needling. When injecting into the trigger point of the supraspinous tendon, meticulously sterile conditions should be observed owing to the close proximity of the joint. The muscle is stretched by adducting and maximally rotating the upper arm inward, while simultaneously rotating the arm slightly to the back.

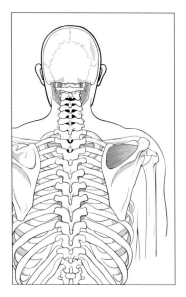

▶ **Fig. 53.1** Supraspinatus muscle.

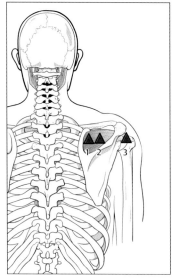

▶ **Fig. 53.2** Trigger points of the supraspinatus muscle.

Trigger Points and Pain Projection Areas

Trigger points 1 and 2: Located in the muscle belly. Trigger point 1 is located at the transition of the acromion to the spine of the scapula. Trigger point 2 is located in the infraspinous fossa close to the origin and the medial margin of the scapula (▶ **Fig. 53.3**). Patients complain about radiating pain, with the main projection areas over the deltoid muscle and also over the head of the radius, and minor pain radiating into the region of the dorsal shoulder girdle, the dorsolateral and ventral upper and lower arm.

Trigger point 3: Located in the supraspinous tendon, with the main pain projection area over the deltoid muscle.
  ▶ **Fig. 53.4**

Important Acupuncture Points

▶ Fig. 53.5

SI-12

Location: Cranial to SI-11, approximately 1 Cun above the middle of the cranial border of the spine of the scapula.

SI-13

Location: Right above the spine of the scapula, in the middle of the connecting line between SI-10 and the spinous process (lower pole) of T2.

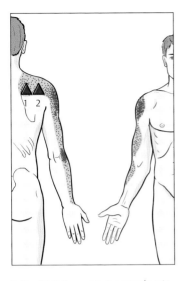

▶ **Fig. 53.3** Supraspinatus muscle, trigger points 1 and 2.

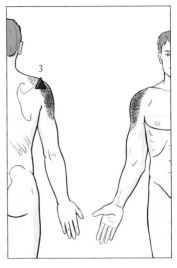

▶ **Fig. 53.4** Supraspinatus muscle, trigger point 3.

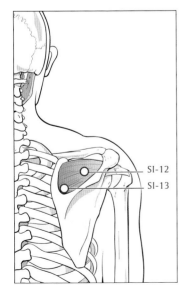

▶ **Fig. 53.5** SI-12 and 13.

54 Infraspinatus Muscle

Description of the Muscle

▶ Fig. 54.1

Origin: Infraspinous fossa of the scapula.

Insertion: Middle and lower third of the greater tubercle of the humerus, joint capsule.

Innervation: Suprascapular nerve (C4–C6).

Action:
- Outward rotation
- Upper part: abduction
- Lower part: adduction

Note: The infraspinatus muscle belongs to the muscles of the rotator cuff because it extends into the capsule of the shoulder joint.

Trigger Points

Introduction: This area predominantly contains two trigger points. A third trigger point inconstantly appears at the medial margin at the level of the middle of the infraspinous fossa. These trigger points are activated by unaccustomed physical activities such as sports (e.g., excessive tennis playing). Differential diagnosis should consider structural disorders of the shoulder joint, stiffness of the shoulder and affections of the nerve roots at C5, C6, and C7.

Examination of trigger points: Provocation is achieved by abducting the arm and maximally rotating it inward in the shoulder joint to stretch the infraspinatus muscle. When the arms are relaxed, typical taut bands are located caudal to the spine of the scapula.

Trigger point therapy: Targeted needling of trigger points and releasing muscular contraction by dry-needling. Therapeutic local anesthesia is also possible. This is followed by passive stretching of the muscles through retroversion and internal rotation of the arm.

Trigger Points and Pain Projection Areas

Trigger points 1 and 2: Both trigger points are located in the

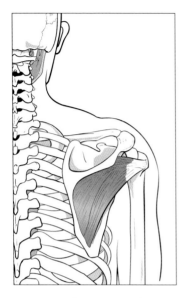

▶ **Fig. 54.1** Infraspinatus muscle.

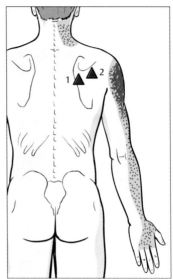

▶ **Fig. 54.2** Infraspinatus muscle, trigger points 1 and 2.

medial half of the muscle, approximately 2 Cun below the scapular spine. Their pain projection areas are over the dorsal as well as ventral portions of the deltoid muscle, with radiation into the dorsal and ventral upper and lower arm on the radial side (▶ Fig. 54.2).

Trigger point 3: Located at the mediocaudal origin, with its area of pain projection at the medial margin of the scapula (▶ **Fig. 54.3**, ▶ **Fig. 54.4**). It appears only inconstantly.

Important Acupuncture Points

▶ **Fig. 54.5**

SI-10

Location: Right above SI-9, below the easily palpable scapular spine.

SI-11

Location: In the infraspinous fossa, on the connecting line between the middle of the easily palpable scapular spine and the inferior angle of the scapula. SI-11 is located between the cranial third and the other two-thirds of this line.

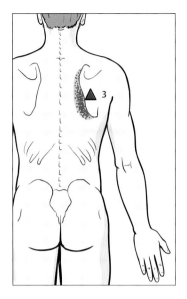

▶ **Fig. 54.3** Infraspinatus muscle, trigger point 3 (1).

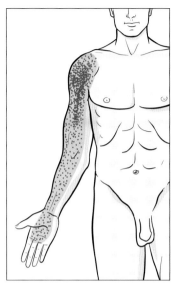

▶ **Fig. 54.4** Infraspinatus muscle, trigger point 3 (2).

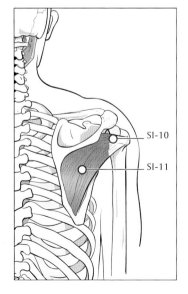

▶ **Fig. 54.5** SI-10 and 11.

55 Subscapular Muscle

Description of the Muscle

▶ Fig. 55.1

Origin: Subscapular fossa of the scapula (not at the neck of the scapula).

Insertion: Lesser tubercle of the humerus and proximal crest of the lesser tubercle.

Innervation: Subscapular nerve (C5/C6).

Action: Inward rotation; tightens the joint capsule into which the subscapular muscle also extends (muscle of the rotator cuff).

Trigger Points

Introduction: There are three trigger points in this area; however, they are difficult to access for treatment because of the location of the muscle. Trigger points of this muscle usually appear as a result of chronic changes, which are generally subsumed under the term "frozen shoulder." The trigger points of the subscapular muscle usually appear in combination with those of the greater pectoral muscle, teres major muscle, latissimus dorsi muscle, and the long head of the triceps muscle.

Examination of trigger points: With patients lying on their back and slight traction of the arm with approximately 90° abduction and internal rotation, palpate the anterior side of the scapula medially to the latissimus dorsi muscle using the thumb of the other hand. Local twitch responses can be triggered in the region of the activated trigger points.

Trigger point therapy: Targeted needling, dry-needling and therapeutic local anesthesia may be applied. However, this requires significantly longer needles and injection needles (approx. 7–8 cm in length). Treatment is followed by stretching the muscle by external rotation and up to 90° abduction, which can be successively increased up to 180° abduction. These physiotherapeutic methods are supported by postisometric relaxation.

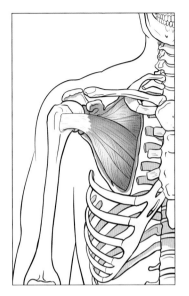

▶ **Fig. 55.1** Subscapular muscle.

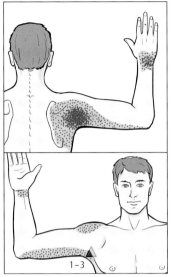

▶ **Fig. 55.2** Subscapular muscle, trigger points 1 to 3.

Trigger Points and Pain Projection Areas

Trigger points 1 to 3: Located in the cranial and middle third of the muscle. They share pain projection areas at the dorsal upper arm, including the scapula, over the deltoid muscle, as well as the dorsal and ventral aspects of the wrist (▶ **Fig. 55.2**).

Important Acupuncture Points

Due to its situation (on the inner side of the scapula), this muscle is anatomically inaccessible to direct acupuncture.

56 Supinator Muscle

Description of the Muscle

▶ Fig. 56.1

Origin: Lateral epicondyle of the humerus, supinator crest of the ulna, annular ligament of the radius and collateral radial ligament.
Insertion: Proximal third of the radius (broad-based).
Innervation: Deep branch of the radial nerve from nerve root C5 to C6.
Action: Supinates the elbow joint.

Trigger Points

Introduction: Most trigger points in this area develop as a result of chronic strain from unaccustomed work, for example, driving screws. The resulting contraction of the supinator muscle is among the most common causes of pain in the radial epicondyle of the humerus. This muscle contraction leads to entrapment neuropathy due to compression of the radial nerve in the supinator cleft.

Examination of trigger points: This muscle is easy to palpate with the patient's forearm supine and the elbow joint slightly flexed.

Trigger point therapy: The supinator cleft must be clearly identified to prevent damage to the radial nerve. Manual trigger point treatment may be preferred in this location. Anatomically experienced therapists may perform targeted infiltration or dry-needling of the trigger point. Stretching is done by pronation of the forearm.

Trigger Points and Pain Projection Areas

The main trigger point is usually located in the radial part of the muscle. The pain radiates predominantly into the radial epicondyle of the humerus, but also into the anterior head of the radius in the cubital fossa and into the first dorsal interosseous muscle between the first and second metacarpal bones (▶ Fig. 56.2, ▶ Fig. 56.3).

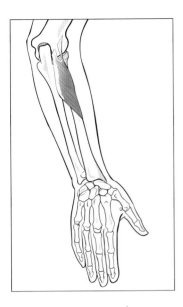

▶ **Fig. 56.1** Supinator muscle.

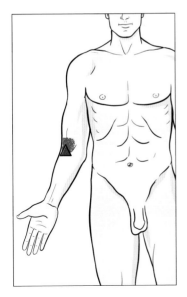

▶ **Fig. 56.2** Supinator muscle, trigger points and pain projection areas (1).

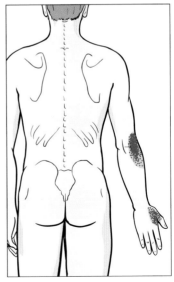

▶ **Fig. 56.3** Supinator muscle, trigger points and pain projection areas (2).

Important Acupuncture Points

▶ Fig. 56.4

LI-8

Location: If the line connecting LI-5 and LI-11 is divided into three equal parts, LI-8 is located two-thirds proximal to LI-5 and one-third distal to LI-11; LI-8 is located 4 Cun distal to LI-11.

LI-9

Location: 3 Cun distal to LI-11.

LI-10

Location: 2 Cun distal to LI-11, on a line connecting LI-5 and LI-11, in the long radial extensor muscle of the wrist (in the supinator muscle, if needled more deeply).

LI-11

Location: Lateral to the radial end of the elbow flexion crease, with the forearm flexed at a right angle, in a depression between the end of the crease and the lateral epicondyle in the area of the long radial extensor muscle of the wrist. LI-11 is located between LU-5 and the lateral epicondyle of the humerus.

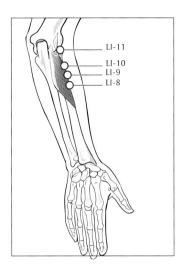

► **Fig. 56.4** LI-8, 9, 10, and 11.

57 Long Radial Extensor Muscle of the Wrist

Description of the Muscle

▶ Fig. 57.1

Origin: Lateral supraepicondylar ridge of the humerus in distal third.

Insertion: Base of second metacarpal bone.

Innervation: Deep branch of the radial nerve (C6/C7).

Action: Extension and radial abduction in the wrist.

Trigger Points

Introduction: This area contains one main trigger point zone. Trigger points in this region are common. Activation usually occurs due to muscular imbalance between the extensor and flexor muscles of the lower arm. Associated trigger points are located in the extensor muscle of the fingers, supinator muscle, and brachioradial muscle.

Examination of trigger points: With the patient's wrist slightly flexed and fingers flexed, vigorous local twitch responses can be triggered quite frequently by direct palpation of the respective muscle. Trigger points can also be quickly diagnosed by isometric testing using a fractionated examination technique.

Trigger point therapy: Conventional acupuncture and therapeutic local anesthesia as well as targeted intramuscular stimulation using acupuncture needles are extremely successful. Passive stretching of the muscles—supported by postisometric relaxation, if necessary—to prevent relapses.

Trigger Points and Pain Projection Areas

Trigger point 1: Located in the muscle belly at the level of the head of the radius. Its pain projection areas are over the head of the radius and dorsally over the abductor muscle of the thumb (▶ Fig. 57.2).

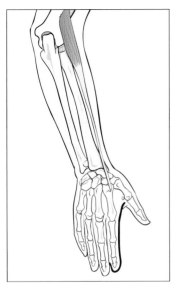

▶ **Fig. 57.1** Long radial extensor muscle of the wrist.

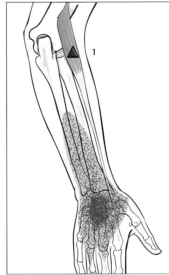

▶ **Fig. 57.2** Long radial extensor muscle of the wrist, trigger point 1.

Important Acupuncture Points

▶ Fig. 57.3

LI-8

Location: On the connecting line between LI-5 and LI-11, two-thirds proximal to LI-5 and one-third distal to LI-11; LI-8 is 4 Cun distal to LI-11.

LI-9

Location: 3 Cun distal to LI-11.

LI-10

Location: 2 Cun distal to LI-11.

LI-11

Location: With lower arm flexed at a right angle, lateral to the radial end of the elbow flexion crease, in a depression between the end of the crease and the lateral epicondyle, in the region of the long radial extensor muscle of the wrist. This point is located between LU-5 and the lateral epicondyle of the humerus.

LI-12

Location: 1 Cun obliquely above LI-11, close to the humerus.

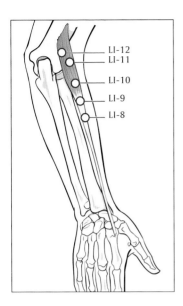

▶ **Fig. 57.3** LI-8, 9, 10, 11, and 12.

58 Extensor Muscle of the Fingers

Description of the Muscle

▶ Fig. 58.1

Origin: Lateral epicondyle of the humerus, annular and collateral ligaments of the radius, fascia of the lower arm.

Insertion: Dorsal aponeurosis. Proximal to the middle finger joints, the aponeurosis divides into the ulnar and radial tendinous portions, which reunite distally to the joint in an aponeurosis and insert at the base of the terminal phalanges.

Innervation: Deep branch of the radial nerve (C6–C8).

Action: Extends finger joints, extends wrist and supports ulnar abduction.

Trigger Points

Introduction: The trigger points are located predominantly in the muscle bellies of the ring and middle finger extensors. Activation of these trigger points usually results from chronic strain. Associated trigger points are often also present in the finger muscles and the extensor muscle of the wrist.

Examination of trigger points: Typical local twitch responses can be triggered in the middle of the muscle belly in the region of these trigger points.

Trigger point therapy: Quick results can be achieved through targeted intramuscular stimulation, with subsequent passive stretching of the muscle. Conventional needling and therapeutic local anesthesia may also be considered.

Trigger Points and Pain Projection Areas

Trigger point 1: The trigger point of the middle finger extensor is located close to the elbow in the region of the muscle belly. Typical pain projection runs along the muscle into the middle finger; sometimes, pain is also localized over the proximal flexion crease of the wrist (▶ Fig. 58.2).

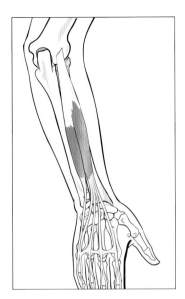

▶ **Fig. 58.1** Extensor muscle of the fingers.

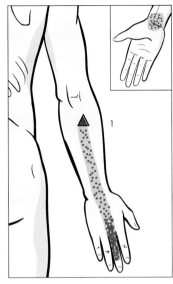

▶ **Fig. 58.2** Extensor muscle of the fingers, trigger point 1.

Trigger point 2: The trigger point of the ring finger extensor is located distal and ulnar to trigger point 1. Its area of pain projection reaches into the ring finger and up toward the radiohumeral joint (▶ Fig. 58.3).

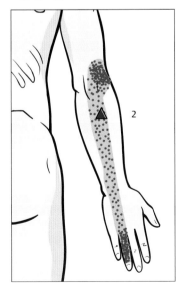

▶ **Fig. 58.3** Extensor muscle of the fingers, trigger point 2.

Important Acupuncture Points

► Fig. 58.4, ► Fig. 58.5

LI-8

Location: 4 Cun distal to LI-11.

LI-9

Location: 3 Cun distal to LI-11.

LI-10

Location: 2 Cun distal to LI-11.

LI-11

Location: With the lower arm flexed at a right angle, lateral to the radial end of the elbow flexion crease, in a depression between the end of the crease and the lateral epicondyle, in the region of the long radial extensor of the wrist.

TE-4

Location: Slightly ulnar to the center of the dorsal flexion crease of the wrist (the joint space between radius, ulna, and proximal wrist bone series), ulnar to the tendon of the extensor muscle of the fingers, and radial to the tendon of the extensor muscle of the little finger.

TE-5

Location: 2 Cun proximal to TE-4, slightly ulnar to the dorsal flexion crease of the wrist (see TE-4 above), on a line connecting TE-4 and the tip of the olecranon process, between the radius and ulna.

TE-6

Location: 3 Cun proximal to TE-4 (location of TE-4: slightly ulnar to the middle of the dorsal wrist flexion crease), between the radius and ulna, on a line connecting TE-4 and the tip of the olecranon (see also info for TE-5 above).

TE-8

Location: 4 Cun proximal to TE-4 (see also TE-4 above), slightly ulnar to the dorsal wrist flexion crease, between the radius and ulna.

TE-9

Location: 7 Cun proximal to TE-4, on a line connecting TE-4 and the tip of the olecranon. On this connecting line, TE-9 is located 1 Cun proximal to the middle between TE-4 and the elbow flexion crease.

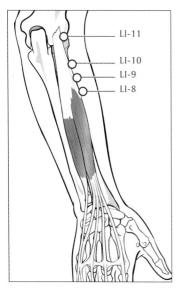

▶ **Fig. 58.4** LI-8, 9, 10, and 11.

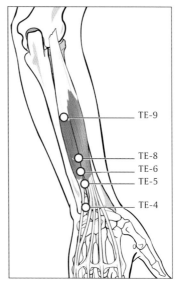

▶ **Fig. 58.5** TE-4, 5, 6, 8, and 9.

59 Pronator Teres Muscle

Description of the Muscle

▶ Fig. 59.1
Origin:
- Humeral head: medial epicondyle of the humerus
- Ulnar head: coronoid process of the ulna

Insertion: Lateral surface of the middle radius and pronator tuberosity.

Innervation: Median nerve from the nerve root C6 to C7.

Action: Pronates the forearm, weak flexor for elbow joint.

Trigger Points

Introduction: These trigger points are usually located in the proximal part of the muscle belly. They are activated by frequent, excessive pronation of the forearm, either through excessive physical work or through chronic stress from sports (e.g., amateur tennis player with poor serve technique).

Since the median nerve passes underneath and sometimes through the pronator teres muscle, it can become compressed. This may lead to a characteristic entrapment neuropathy that may ultimately resemble carpal tunnel syndrome.

Examination of trigger points: This muscle is easy to examine by deep palpation in the cubital fossa. Palpation triggers the characteristic radiation of pain.

Trigger point therapy: There is a risk of damaging the median nerve. Before dry-needling or injecting the trigger points, the course of the median nerve must be precisely identified. Manual treatment using acupressure is another option.

Trigger Points and Pain Projection Areas

Trigger point 1: This is the main trigger point and is located in the muscle belly in the cubital fossa, near the origin of the muscle. The pain radiates from the proximal anteroradial part of the forearm to the wrist, where it reaches the proximal palmar part of the thumb (▶ Fig. 59.2).

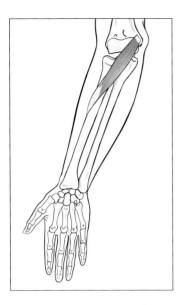

▶ **Fig. 59.1** Pronator teres muscle.

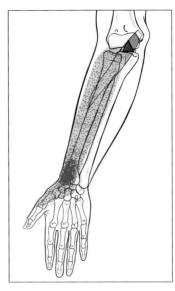

▶ **Fig. 59.2** Pronator teres muscle, trigger point 1.

Important Acupuncture Points

▶ Fig. 59.3

PC-3

Location: On the ulnar side of the tendon of the biceps muscle of the arm, in the elbow flexion crease.

HT-3

Location: With elbow flexed, between the ulnar end of the elbow flexion crease and the medial epicondyle of the humerus.

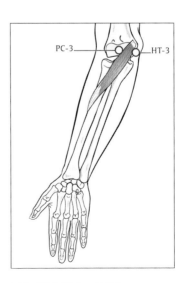

▶ **Fig. 59.3** PC-3 and HT-3.

60 Superficial Flexor Muscle of the Fingers

▶ Fig. 60.1

Description of the Muscle

Origin:
- Humeroulnar head: medial epicondyle of the humerus and coronoid process of the ulna
- Radial head: anterior surface of the radius

Insertion: Four tendons insert on the lateral bony ridges of the middle phalanges from the index finger to the little finger.

Innervation: Median nerve from nerve root C7 to T1.

Action: The muscle flexes the second to fifth metacarpophalangeal joints and second to fifth proximal interphalangeal joints.

Trigger Points

Introduction: The flexors of the fingers, like the tensors of the fingers, are deemed to be superficial muscles. However, they are covered by the ulnar and radial flexor muscles of the wrist. To avoid damage to the nerves, deep needling should never be performed. Trigger point activation is caused by chronic strain, especially due to manual labor. In particular, monotonous grasping movements activate these trigger points.

Examination of trigger points: It requires only slight pressure to palpate the trigger points in the middle of the muscle belly. This is done by gently palpating through the ulnar and radial flexor muscles of the wrist as well as the palmar muscle. Precise identification is confirmed by increased sensation of pain when palpating the trigger points while simultaneously performing muscle function tests.

Trigger point therapy: Careful dry-needling or injection can prevent damage to the nerve structures of the median nerve, ulnar artery, and ulnar nerve. These trigger points are easy to

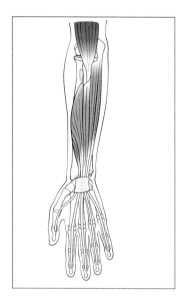

▶ **Fig. 60.1** Superficial flexor muscle of the fingers.

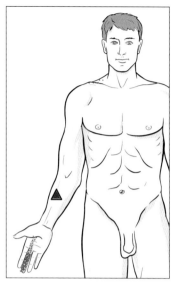

▶ **Fig. 60.2** Trigger points and pain projection areas (1).

inactivate. Subsequent stretching of the flexors by dorsal extension of the fingers is essential for preventing relapses, and patients can do these exercises on their own.

Trigger Points and Pain Projection Areas

In the radial portion of the flexor muscles, the pain radiates into the palmar side of the middle finger; in the ulnar portion, it radiates into the ring finger or little finger (▶ Fig. 60.2), sometimes with further projection into the palm (▶ Fig. 60.3).

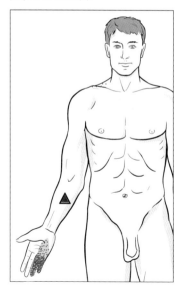

▶ **Fig. 60.3** Trigger points and pain projection areas (2).

Important Acupuncture Points

▶ Fig. 60.4

LU-5

Location: Radial to the biceps tendons in the elbow flexion crease.

LU-7

Location: On the radial side of the forearm, in a **V**-shaped groove proximal to the styloid process of the radius, 1.5 Cun proximal to the wrist flexion crease. LU-7 is located where the proximal portion of the styloid process of the radius merges into the shaft of the radius.

PC-3

Location: On the ulnar side of the tendon of the biceps muscle of the arm in the elbow flexion crease.

PC-6

Location: 2 Cun proximal to the wrist flexion crease, proximal to the pisiform bone, between the tendons of the palmaris longus muscle and the radial flexor muscle of the wrist.

PC-7

Location: In the middle of the wrist flexion crease, proximal to the pisiform bone, between the tendons of the palmaris longus muscle and the radial flexor muscle of the wrist.

HT-3

Location: With elbow flexed, between the ulnar end of the elbow flexion crease and the medial epicondyle of the humerus.

HT-4

Location: 1.5 Cun proximal to HT-7, radial to the tendon of the ulnar flexor muscle of the wrist.

HT-5

Location: 1 Cun proximal to HT-7, radial to the tendon of the ulnar flexor muscle of the wrist.

HT-7

Location: At the wrist flexion crease, radial to the tendon of the ulnar flexor muscle of the wrist.

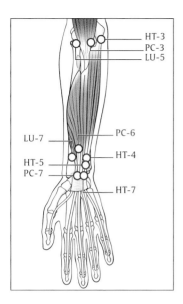

▶ **Fig. 60.4** LU-5, 7, PC-3, 6, 7, HT-3, 4, 5, and 7.

61   External Oblique Muscle of the Abdomen

Description of the Muscle

▶ Fig. 61.1

Origin: Inferior borders and outer surfaces of the 5th to 12th ribs.

Insertion: Pubic tubercle, pubic crest, outer margin of iliac crest, inguinal ligament, and white line (linea alba).

Innervation: Intercostal nerves (T5–T11), subcostal nerve from nerve root T12, iliohypogastric nerve (T12–L1) and ilioinguinal nerve from nerve root L1.

Action: Rotates the thorax against the pelvis to the contralateral side. Bilateral contraction flexes the vertebral column. Auxiliary muscle for abdominal compression, simultaneous action as auxiliary respiratory muscle for forced expiration.

Trigger Points of the External Oblique Muscle of the Abdomen

Introduction: These trigger points frequently develop in connection with acute abdomen (boardlike, hard abdomen). Trigger points are also observed with disorders of the inner organs, such as dysmenorrhea, diarrhea, spasm of the urinary bladder, and testicular pain. These trigger points may occur first and then cause secondary abdominal symptoms. More often, however, the reverse happens: visceral afferent stimuli cause trigger points in the abdominal muscles. Trigger points in the oblique abdominal muscles are frequently associated with acute lumbago.

Examination of trigger points: With the patient seated, taut bands and trigger points in this muscle are provoked by rotating movements.

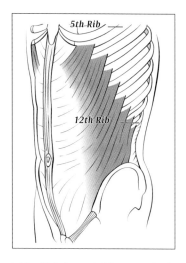

▶ **Fig. 61.1** External oblique muscle of the abdomen.

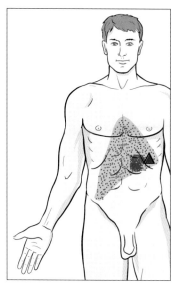

▶ **Fig. 61.2** External oblique muscle of the abdomen, trigger point 1.

Trigger point therapy: Dry-needling is possible in this area without problems, and trigger point infiltration is also an option. Injection or acupuncture of the trigger points is performed with the patient in a supine position. Puncture of the peritoneum must be avoided. However, damage to the inner organs rarely occurs.

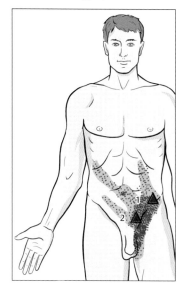

▶ **Fig. 61.3** External oblique muscle of the abdomen, trigger point 2.

Trigger Points and Pain Projection Areas

Trigger Point 1: Located on the anterior border of the costal arch, toward the epigastrium (▶ Fig. 61.2). Its characteristic radiation of pain into the epigastrium can mimic symptoms of angina pectoris or epigastric disorders.

Trigger Point 2: Located near the muscle insertion on the iliac crest. Pain radiates into the groin and into the labia or testes (▶ Fig. 61.3). Prolonged standing causes additional radiation of pain into the entire abdominal region, which makes it difficult to locate the primary origin.

Important Acupuncture Points

▶ Fig. 61.4

CV-2

Location: At the superior border of the pubic symphysis, on the anterior median line.

CV-3

Location: 1 Cun cranial to the middle of the superior border of the pubic symphysis.

CV-4

Location: 2 Cun cranial to the middle of the superior border of the pubic symphysis. (For precise orientation, see also CV-3 above.)

CV-6

Location: 1.5 Cun inferior to the umbilicus. (For precise orientation, see also CV-3 above.)

CV-12

Location: Midway between the base of the xiphoid process and the umbilicus.

CV-14

Location: 1 Cun caudal to the tip of the xiphoid process (CV-15).

CV-15

Location: Just below the tip of the xiphoid process, on the anterior median line.

LR-13

Location: At the free end of the 11th rib.

LR-14

Location: In the sixth intercostal space, below the nipple, on the mammillary line.

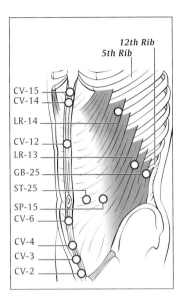

▶ **Fig. 61.4** CV-2, 3, 4, 6, 12, 14, 15, LR-13, 14, ST-25, SP-15, and GB-25.

ST-25

Location: 2 Cun lateral to the umbilicus.

SP-15

Location: 4 Cun lateral to the umbilicus.

GB-25

Location: At the free end of the 12th rib.

62 Iliac Muscle / Psoas Muscle

The iliac muscle merges with the greater psoas muscle into the iliopsoas muscle.

Description of the Iliac Muscle

▶ Fig. 62.1

Origin: The entire iliac fossa to the terminal line of the pelvis, anterior inferior iliac spine, and lacuna of muscles to anterior surface of the hip joint capsule.

Insertion: Lesser trochanter of the femur.

Innervation: Femoral nerve, T12 to L3/L4.

Action: With pelvic and lumbar regions fixed, strongest flexor muscle of the hip joint (iliopsoas muscle), together with the greater psoas muscle. With the femur immobilized, it rotates the ipsilateral pelvis laterally.

Trigger Points of the Iliac Muscle

Introduction: Muscle contractions are very commonly observed with coxarthrosis. This muscle has a general tendency to contract and develop trigger points (▶ Fig. 62.2). This tendency is often significantly increased by visceral afferent stimuli occurring in response to irritation of the cecum directly bordering the fascia of the iliac muscle. Trigger points in this area frequently appear in association with trigger points of other muscles (quadratus lumborum, rectus abdominis and rectus femoris, tensor fascia lata). Treatment of these secondary trigger points is therefore recommended.

Examination of trigger points: With the patient relaxed in a supine position, the muscle can be directly palpated between the cecum and the inside of the iliac bone. However, adhesions in this area often make this difficult and require manual mobilization of the cecum before proceeding. One trigger point is located in the more anterior part of the muscle. Another trigger point is located at the level of the actual hip joint.

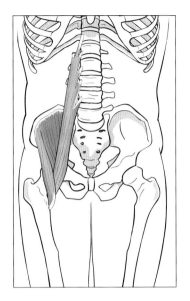

▶ **Fig. 62.1** Iliac muscle.

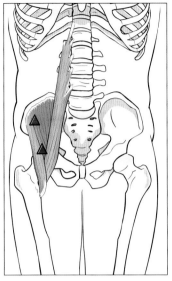

▶ **Fig. 62.2** Trigger points of the iliac muscle.

Trigger point therapy: Acupuncture of the trigger points in the iliac muscle may be attempted if the cecum can be moved far enough in a medial direction. It is important to treat the cause of the visceral lesion as well. Relapses are prevented by physiotherapeutic stretching involving extension of the ipsilateral hip joint, with simultaneous maximum flexion of the contralateral hip joint and stretching of the rectus femoris muscle, which is usually also shortened.

Description of the Psoas Muscle

▶ Fig. 62.3

Origin: Lateral surfaces of vertebrae T12 and L1 to L4, the adjoining intervertebral disks and the costal processes of the lumbar vertebrae.

Insertion: Lesser trochanter of the femur.

Innervation: Femoral nerve, T12 to L3/L4.

Action: Together with the iliac muscle, strongest flexor muscle of the hip joint (iliopsoas muscle). With the femur fixed, it flexes the lumbar spine, posteriorly rotates the ipsilateral half of the pelvis and laterally flexes the lumbar spine.

ⓘ Additional Information

The lumbar plexus is located between the two portions of the psoas muscle.

Trigger Points of the Psoas Muscle

Introduction: The psoas muscle is subdivided into the smaller psoas muscle and the greater psoas muscle. Trigger points are frequently located in the region of the greater psoas muscle (▶ **Fig. 62.4**). They are associated with chronic strain injuries, poor muscular posture of the lumbar spine, and coxarthrosis. Visceral afferent stimuli also play a role here. They originate from the kidneys, which directly overlay the psoas muscle, or from the traversing sigmoid colon on the left. Anterior iliac lesions are therefore frequently located on the right (with anterior rotation of the pelvic half) and posterior iliac lesions are located on the left (with posterior rotation of the pelvic half). This results in a functional difference in leg length caused by a shortening of the left leg or a lengthening of the right leg, due to distal displacement (on the right) or proximal displacement (on the left) of the rotational center of the hip joint. It is, therefore, always recommended to treat not only the trigger points but also the causes of the underlying distortion of the pelvis.

Examination of trigger points: The greater psoas muscle can only be examined in a relaxed patient and by using deep palpation. This muscle is often very sensitive to pressure. Jump signs are absent.

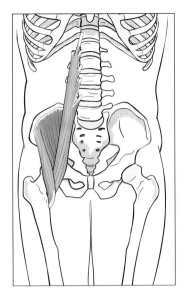

▶ **Fig. 62.3** Psoas muscle.

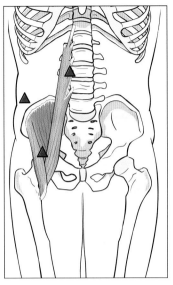

▶ **Fig. 62.4** Trigger points of the psoas muscle.

Trigger point therapy: Trigger points in the region of the psoas muscle are usually not at all or poorly accessible to dry-needling or injection. Other stretching methods are therefore recommended, such as myofascial release.

Trigger Points and Pain Projection Areas

Iliopsoas Muscle

▶ Fig. 62.5, ▶ Fig. 62.6

Trigger points 1 to 3: Trigger point 1 is located in the ventral portion of the iliopsoas muscle and prevertebrally at the level of vertebra L3. Trigger point 2 is located directly above the hip joint. Trigger point 3 is located at the iliac muscle. Their pain projection areas are directly paravertebral in the lumbar region, with radiation into the sacroiliac joint and the upper medial gluteal area. Another pain projection area appears over the rectus femoris muscle, with radiation toward the anterior superior iliac spine.

Important Acupuncture Points

This muscle is anatomically inaccessible to direct acupuncture.

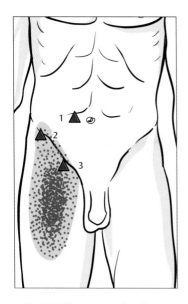

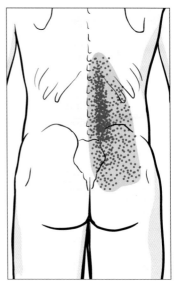

▶ **Fig. 62.5** Iliopsoas muscle, trigger points 1 to 3 (1).

▶ **Fig. 62.6** Iliopsoas muscle, trigger points 1 to 3 (2).

63 Quadratus Lumborum Muscle

Description of the Muscle

▶ Fig. 63.1

Origin:
- Dorsal fibers: iliac crest and iliolumbar ligament
- Ventral parts: costal processes of vertebrae L2 to L5

Insertion:
- Dorsal part: 12th rib and costal processes of vertebrae L1 to L3
- Ventral part: 12th rib

Innervation: Subcostal nerve and lumbar plexus (T12–L3).

Action: Flexes the trunk laterally, stabilizes the 12th rib during respiration (fixed point for the diaphragm).

Trigger Points

Introduction: This muscle contains four trigger points (▶ Fig. 63.2), two each in the deep and superficial portions of the muscle. Disorders of the sacroiliac joint frequently present clinically. Activation of trigger points results from acute strain, also in connection with accidents and from chronic strain in functional scoliosis (as a result of unequal leg lengths) or in primary scoliosis. Associated trigger points appear in the region of the abdominal muscles, contralateral quadratus lumborum muscle, ipsilateral iliac/psoas muscle and iliocostal muscle; occasionally also in the latissimus dorsi muscle and internal oblique muscle of the abdomen. Additional trigger points are located in the gluteal region, especially with symptoms of nerve root irritation related to nerve roots L5 and S1.

Examination of trigger points: The first step is to clarify the following orthopedic causes: functional or structural scoliosis, obliquity of the pelvis, and pelvic distortion. Successful palpation of trigger points is achieved in patients lying relaxed on their side. Local twitch responses are rarely observed. Usually, there is distinct hardening of the muscle.

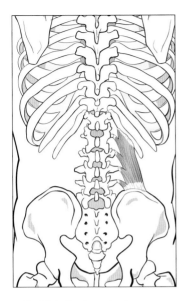

▶ **Fig. 63.1** Quadratus lumborum muscle.

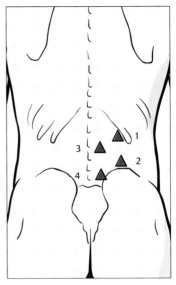

▶ **Fig. 63.2** Trigger points of the quadratus lumborum muscle.

Trigger point therapy: Direct needling is only possible with acupuncture needles of at least 60 mm in length. Therapeutic local anesthesia is a possible alternative. Dry-needling can usually be successfully performed as well; in a lateral position, the needle is aimed in the direction of the transverse processes. Follow-up treatment involves stretching of the muscles using postisometric relaxation by adduction of the hip joint, with patients lying on their back with their hip joint flexed approximately 80°. This also stretches the entire gluteal region.

Trigger Points and Pain Projection Areas

Trigger points 1 and 2: The superficial trigger point 1 (▶ Fig. 63.3, ▶ Fig. 63.4) is located approximately 2 Cun below the lateral end of the muscle border and 2 Cun below the 12th rib. Its pain projection area is at the level of the lateral and dorsal proximal gluteal regions, with radiation toward the groin and the sacroiliac joint. Trigger point 2 (▶ Fig. 63.3, ▶ Fig. 63.4) is located at the level of L4, just above the insertion of the quadratus lumborum muscle, at the dorsolateral iliac crest. Its pain projection area is at the level of the greater trochanter and radiates in ventral and dorsal directions.

Trigger points 3 and 4: These trigger points of the muscle's deep portion (▶ Fig. 63.5) are located at the level of L3 and L4. Their typical pain projection areas are over the sacroiliac joint and in the lower middle of the buttock.

Important Acupuncture Points

▶ Fig. 63.6

BL-23

Location: 1.5 Cun lateral to the lower edge of the spinous process of vertebra L2.

BL-51

Location: 3 Cun lateral to the lower edge of the spinous process of vertebra L1.

BL-52

Location: 3 Cun lateral to the lower edge of the spinous process of vertebra L2.

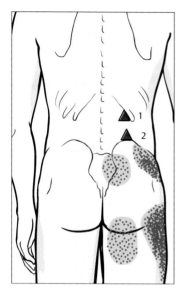

▶ **Fig. 63.3** Quadratus lumborum muscle, trigger points 1 and 2 (1).

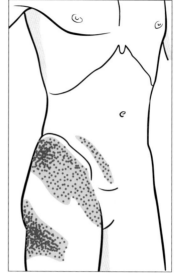

▶ **Fig. 63.4** Quadratus lumborum muscle, trigger points 1 and 2 (2).

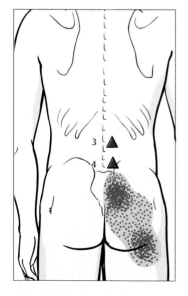

▶ **Fig. 63.5** Quadratus lumborum muscle, trigger points 3 and 4.

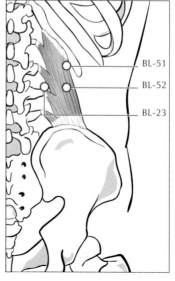

▶ **Fig. 63.6** BL-23, 51, and 52.

64 Gluteus Maximus Muscle

Description of the Muscle

▶ Fig. 64.1

Origin: Dorsal aspect of the ilium, thoracolumbar fascia, lateral edge of the sacrum and coccyx, sacrotuberal ligament.

Insertion: Gluteal tuberosity of the femur, iliotibial tract of the fascia lata, lateral intermuscular septum.

Innervation: Inferior gluteal nerve (L4–S1).

Action: Extension in the hip joint: upper fibers, abduction; lower fibers, adduction and rotation of the thigh laterally.

Trigger Points

Introduction: This muscle contains three trigger points. Trigger points in this region often appear in combination with trigger points of the gluteus minimus muscle and the sciaticocrural muscle. Trigger points of the deep erector muscles of the spine are also found to be associated. Activation often results from acute events associated with increased strain of the gluteus maximus muscle. Such trigger points are frequently found in athletes.

Examination of trigger points: These trigger points are superficially located and can be easily palpated. Local twitch responses are rarely observed. Especially for trigger points 1 and 2, direct pressure sensibility of the sciatic nerve in the sense of Valleix points should be differentiated.

Trigger point therapy: Inactivation of these trigger points is achieved without any problems by acupuncture, dry-needling, and therapeutic local anesthesia. Targeted stretching exercises using postisometric relaxation completes the treatment.

Trigger Points and Pain Projection Areas

Trigger point 1: Trigger point 1 (▶ Fig. 64.2) is located on the extension of a vertical line through the posterior iliac spine at the level of the proximal end of the anal cleft. Its main projection areas are along the medial and caudal margins of the muscle.

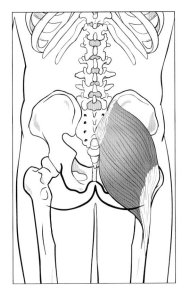

▶ **Fig. 64.1** Gluteus maximus muscle.

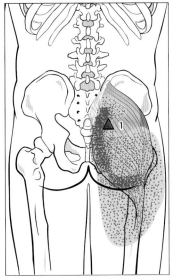

▶ **Fig. 64.2** Gluteus maximus muscle, trigger point 1.

Trigger point 2: Trigger point 2 (▶ Fig. 64.3) is located at the level of the caudal margin of the muscle, approximately 4 to 5 cm above the gluteal fold. Pain projection areas are located in this region, in the entire gluteal region including the region over the caudal sacrum, and above the greater trochanter.

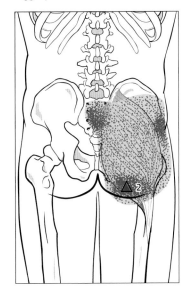

▶ **Fig. 64.3** Gluteus maximus muscle, trigger point 2.

Trigger point 3: Trigger point 3 (▶ **Fig. 64.4**) is located at the mediocaudal margin of the muscle. Its main projection area is in the direction of the coccyx.

Important Acupuncture Points

▶ Fig. 64.5

BL-27

Location: At the level of the first sacral foramen, 1.5 Cun lateral to the posterior median line, in a depression between the sacrum and upper region of the posterior superior iliac spine.

BL-28

Location: At the level of the second sacral foramen, 1.5 Cun lateral to the posterior median line.

BL-29

Location: At the level of the third sacral foramen, 1.5 Cun lateral to the posterior median line.

BL-30

Location: At the level of the fourth sacral foramen, 1.5 Cun lateral to the posterior median line.

BL-36

Location: In the middle of the gluteal fold.

BL-53

Location: At the level of the second sacral foramen, 1.5 Cun lateral to BL-28.

BL-54

Location: At the level of the fourth sacral foramen, 3 Cun lateral to the sacral hiatus.

GB-30

Location: On the lateral side of the hip joint, on a line connecting the greater trochanter and the sacral hiatus, between the outer and middle thirds.

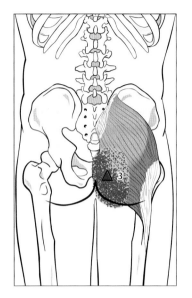

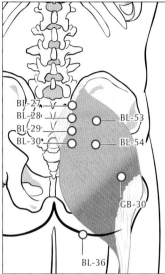

▶ **Fig. 64.4** Gluteus maximus muscle, trigger point 3.

▶ **Fig. 64.5** BL-27, 28, 29, 30, 36, 53, 54, and GB-30.

65 Gluteus Medius Muscle

Description of the Muscle

► Fig. 65.1

Origin: Ala of ilium between the anterior and posterior gluteal lines.
Insertion: Greater trochanter of the femur.
Innervation: Superior gluteal nerve (L4–S1).
Action: Abducts the leg in the hip joint. Stabilizes the pelvis on the side of the supporting leg. Slight contribution to medial rotation of the nonsupporting leg.

Trigger Points

Introduction: These trigger points (► Fig. 65.2) are located along the entire muscle. They develop particularly due to strain caused by sports or work, but also after accidents. Dysfunction of the sacroiliac joint is frequently observed.

Examination of trigger points: These trigger points can be palpated and provoked easily with the hip joint flexed to 90° and adducted. The same position is used for stretching the shortened muscle groups during follow-up treatment.

Trigger point therapy: Targeted intramuscular stimulation with subsequent passive stretching of the muscle is very effective. Manual therapy, including adjustment of the affected sacroiliac joint, should be performed concurrently. Alternatively, conventional needling or therapeutic local anesthesia may be used.

Trigger Points and Pain Projection Areas

Trigger point 1: Trigger point 1 (► Fig. 65.3) is located in the posterior portion of the gluteus medius muscle, near the posterior superior iliac spine; it leads to radiation of pain around the sacroiliac joint.

Trigger point 2: Trigger point 2 (► Fig. 65.4) is located in the middle of the gluteus medius muscle; it leads to radiation of pain in the gluteal region and into the greater trochanter.

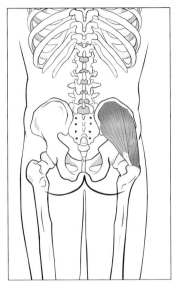

▶ **Fig. 65.1** Gluteus medius muscle.

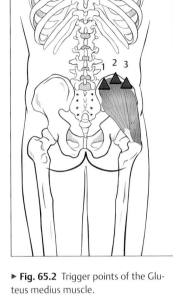

▶ **Fig. 65.2** Trigger points of the Gluteus medius muscle.

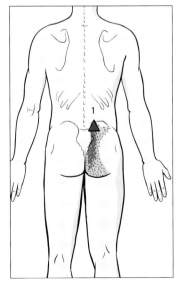

▶ **Fig. 65.3** Gluteus medius muscle, trigger point 1.

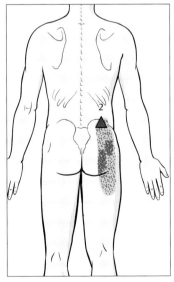

▶ **Fig. 65.4** Gluteus medius muscle, trigger point 2.

Trigger point 3: Trigger point 3 (▶ Fig. 65.5) is located on the anterior border of the muscle; it leads to the characteristic radiation of pain into the ipsilateral sacroiliac joint.

Important Acupuncture Points

▶ Fig. 65.6

EX-B-6

Location: Below the inferior border of the spinous process of vertebra L4, and 3 Cun lateral to the posterior median line.

EX-B-7

Location: 3.5 Cun lateral to the inferior border of the spinous process of vertebra L4.

BL-53

Location: At the level of the second sacral foramen, and 1.5 Cun lateral to BL-28.

BL-54

Location: 3 Cun lateral to the sacral hiatus, at the level of the fourth sacral foramen.

GB-30

Location: On the lateral side of the hip, one-third of the distance between the greater trochanter and the sacral hiatus. In China, this point is always needled with the patient in a lateral position. The hip and knee of the side to be treated are flexed, while the leg beneath is straight.

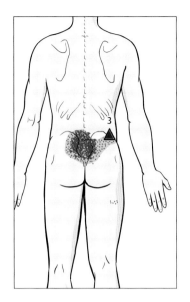

▶ **Fig. 65.5** Gluteus medius muscle, trigger point 3.

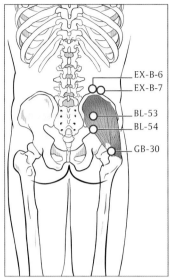

▶ **Fig. 65.6** EX-B-6, EX-B-7, BL-53, 54, and GB-30.

66 Gluteus Minimus Muscle

Description of the Muscle

▶ Fig. 66.1

Origin: Ala of ilium between the anterior and posterior gluteal lines.

Insertion: Greater trochanter of the femur.

Innervation: Superior gluteal nerve from the nerve roots L4 to S1.

Action: When fully contracted, the muscle abducts the thigh. With only the anterior portion of the muscle contracted, it rotates the non-supporting leg medially; with only the posterior portion contracted, it rotates the nonsupporting leg laterally and extends it slightly. Contraction on the side of the supporting leg stabilizes the pelvis.

Trigger Points

Introduction: These trigger points develop quite frequently in combination with those of the gluteus medius. The causes are similar.

Examination of trigger points: The gluteus minimus muscle can only be palpated when the gluteus medius muscle is relaxed; the origin of the gluteus medius is further proximal and superficial. With the patient in the lateral position, palpation is performed with the hip joint flexed to 90° and abducted.

Trigger point therapy: As with the gluteus medius muscle, direct methods such as intramuscular stimulation by dry-needling are very effective when followed by passive stretching with the hip joint flexed and abducted to 90°. Therapeutic local anesthesia or conventional needling is also an option. Patients can also easily stretch these muscles on their own.

Trigger Points and Pain Projection Areas

Trigger points 1: These points (▶ Fig. 66.2) are located in the anterior portion of the muscle. Triggering in this location radiates pain into the posterior gluteal

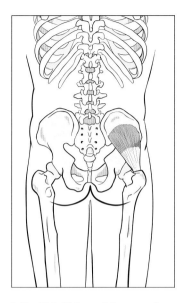

▶ **Fig. 66.1** Gluteus minimus muscle.

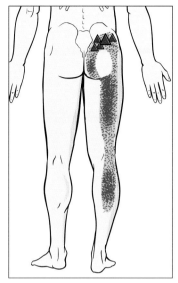

▶ **Fig. 66.3** Gluteus minimus muscle, trigger points 2.

region or along the iliotibial tract, across the knee, and down to the lateral ankle.

Trigger points 2: This group of trigger points (▶ Fig. 66.3) is located more in the medial and posterior portions of the muscle. Triggering in this location radiates pain into the posterior gluteal region and posterolateral thigh down to the posterolateral calf, approximately at the level of the lateral head of the gastrocnemius muscle.

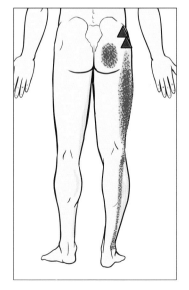

▶ **Fig. 66.2** Gluteus minimus muscle, trigger points 1.

Important Acupuncture Points

▶ Fig. 66.4

BL-53

Location: At the level of the second sacral foramen, 1.5 Cun lateral to BL-28.

BL-54

Location: At the level of the fourth sacral foramen, 3 Cun lateral to the sacral hiatus.

GB-30

Location: On the lateral side of the hip, one-third of the distance on a line between the greater trochanter and the sacral hiatus. In China, this point is always needled with the patient in a lateral position. The hip and knee of the side to be treated are flexed, while the leg beneath is straight.

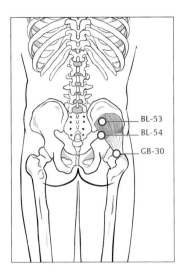

▶ **Fig. 66.4** BL-53, 54, and GB-30.

67 Piriformis Muscle

Description of the Muscle

▶ Fig. 67.1

Origin: Anterior surface of the sacrum.

Insertion: Tip of greater trochanter of the femur.

Innervation: Sacral plexus (L5–S2).

Action: Lateral rotation, abduction.

ℹ Additional Information

In cases of high sciatic nerve division, the common fibular nerve passes across the piriformis muscle and can be constricted there (piriformis syndrome).

Trigger Points

Introduction: The two trigger points of the piriformis muscle are often associated with chronic pain in the loin–pelvis–hip area. They are activated by chronic disorders of the lumbosacral transition and rarely in response to acute strain. In cases where this muscle is shortened, entrapment of the sciatic nerve (especially of the peroneal portion) takes place in approximately 10% due to the aberrant course of the muscle; this should be considered in the differential diagnosis. Active associated trigger points appear regularly in the inferior and superior gemellus muscles, the obturator internus muscle and the gluteus medius and gluteus maximus muscles.

Examination of trigger points: Activation of trigger points is achieved by adducting the hip joint when flexed at 90° and simultaneously counter-rotating the remaining part of the spinal column. The piriformis muscle can be grasped by careful deep palpation between dorsal trochanter and sacrum, with patients lying on their stomach.

Trigger point therapy: These trigger points can be inactivated by conventional acupuncture, dry-needling, and also by therapeutic local anesthesia. Passive stretching supported by postisometric relaxation decisively contributes to treatment success.

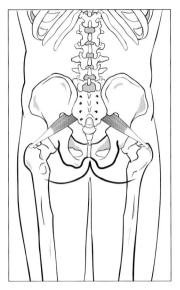

▶ **Fig. 67.1** Piriformis muscle.

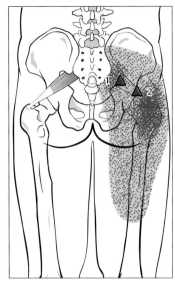

▶ **Fig. 67.2** Piriformis muscle, trigger points 1 and 2.

Trigger Points and Pain Projection Areas

Trigger points 1 and 2: Trigger point 1 is located close to the insertion and has its main area of pain projection dorsal to the greater trochanter. Trigger point 2 is located close to the origin and has its projection area at the caudal pole of the sacroiliac joint. Both points share a common area of radiation over and beyond the buttocks into the dorsal thigh (▶ Fig. 67.2).

Important Acupuncture Points

▶ Fig. 67.3

BL-54

Location: 3 Cun lateral to the sacral hiatus, at the level of the fourth sacral foramen.

GB-30

Location: Lateral side of the hip on a line connecting the greater trochanter and the sacral hiatus, between the outer and middle thirds.

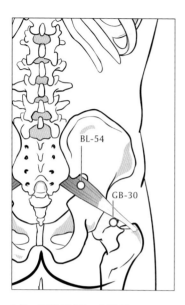

▶ **Fig. 67.3** BL-54 and GB-30.

68 Quadriceps Femoris Muscle

Description of the Muscle

▶ Fig. 68.1, ▶ Fig. 68.2, ▶ Fig. 68.3

Origin:
- Rectus femoris muscle: with one head at the anterior inferior iliac spine, the other at the acetabulum and hip joint capsule
- Vastus medialis muscle: distal part of the intertrochanteric line, medial lip of linea aspera of the femur (rough line of the femur)
- Vastus lateralis muscle: lateral part of greater trochanter, lateral lip of linea aspera of the femur (rough line of the femur), intertrochanteric line
- Vastus intermedius muscle: anterior and lateral surfaces of the femur

Insertion: Base and lateral surface of the patella and tuberosity of the tibia via the patellar ligament.

Innervation: Femoral nerve (L2–L4); indicator muscle for L4.

Action: Extends the knee joint; rectus femoris muscle: flexes the hip joint.

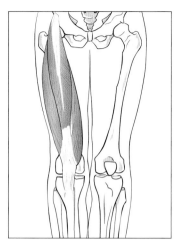

▶ **Fig. 68.1** Quadriceps femoris muscle (1).

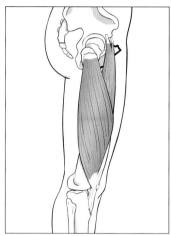

▶ **Fig. 68.2** Quadriceps femoris muscle (2).

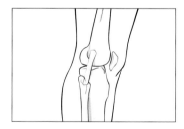

▶ **Fig. 68.3** Quadriceps femoris muscle (3).

Trigger Points

Introduction: Trigger points (▶ Fig. 68.4, ▶ Fig. 68.5) in this group of muscles are very common. Symptoms are mainly restricted to the thigh. Most trigger points are observed in the vastus lateralis muscle. These trigger points are activated by acute strain during sports activities, especially with sudden, intense eccentric contraction. Trigger points in the quadriceps femoris muscle usually appear as a consequence of primary trigger points in the region of the dorsal thigh muscles and soleus muscle. However, primary trigger points can also develop as a result of muscular imbalance between the vastus medialis muscle and the vastus lateralis muscle, when hip and knee joints are affected.

Examination of trigger points: With the hip joint slightly abducted, the rectus femoris muscle is examined by palpating the proximal part using the thumb. The vastus medialis muscle is grasped by direct palpation with the knee flexed and the hip slightly flexed and abducted. During this examination, the knee joint should be supported laterally to avoid the patient actively holding the leg. The vastus intermedius muscle is palpated deeply with the patient lying in the dorsal position, with leg extended and hip and knee joints in neutral positions. Trigger points in the vastus lateralis muscle are also identified by direct palpation, with hip and knee joints slightly flexed and the knee joint supported from below.

Trigger point therapy: Dry-needling seems to be the optimal procedure; typically, this triggers local twitch responses of taut bands. Acupuncture or trigger point infiltration can also be considered. The patient needs to be instructed to stretch the muscles adequately after treatment as they are often shortened. In addition, postisometric relaxation exercises are helpful.

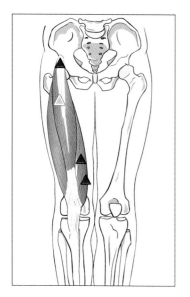 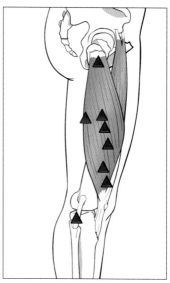

▶ **Fig. 68.4** Trigger points of the quadriceps femoris muscle (1).

▶ **Fig. 68.5** Trigger points of the quadriceps femoris muscle (2).

Trigger Points and Pain Projection Areas

Rectus Femoris Muscle

Trigger point 1: The trigger point of the rectus femoris muscle is located close to the origin of the muscle, directly over the hip joint. It has a typical projection area over the distal anterior thigh (▶ **Fig. 68.6**).

Vastus Intermedius Muscle

Trigger point 1: The vastus intermedius muscle is located below the rectus femoris muscle and contains trigger points in all parts of the muscle. They appear variably and lead to local radiation in the anterior thigh (▶ **Fig. 68.7**).

Vastus Medialis Muscle

Trigger point 1: Trigger point 1 of the vastus medialis muscle is located in the muscle belly, 5 cm proximal to the upper pole of the patella. It leads to radiation symptoms over the medial joint space of the knee and over the distal medial thigh (▶ **Fig. 68.8**).

Trigger point 2: Trigger point 2 of the vastus medialis muscle is located in the middle of the muscle. Its area of pain projection runs along the muscle, predominantly in a distal direction (▶ **Fig. 68.9**).

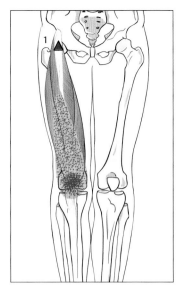

▶ **Fig. 68.6** Quadriceps femoris muscle (rectus femoris muscle), trigger point 1.

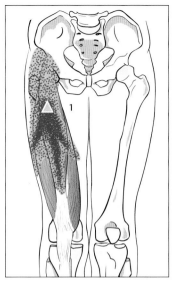

▶ **Fig. 68.7** Quadriceps femoris muscle (vastus intermedius muscle), trigger point 1.

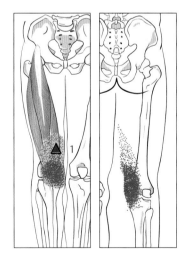

▶ **Fig. 68.8** Quadriceps femoris muscle (vastus medialis muscle), trigger point 1.

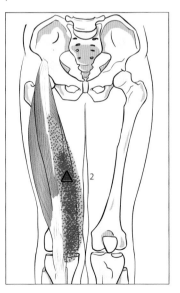

▶ **Fig. 68.9** Quadriceps muscle of the thigh (vastus medialis muscle), trigger point 2.

Vastus Lateralis Muscle

Trigger point 1: Trigger point 1 of the vastus lateralis muscle is located in the ventral part, just above the patella. Its main area of pain projection is laterally around the patella toward the lateral joint space and radiates slightly into the lateral middle portion of the thigh (▶ **Fig. 68.10**).

Trigger point 2: Trigger point 2 of the vastus lateralis muscle is located immediately dorsal to trigger point 1. It radiates into the distal portion of the vastus lateralis muscle, with further projection zones in the dorsolateral thigh and proximal dorsolateral lower leg (▶ **Fig. 68.11**).

Trigger point 3: Trigger point 3 of the vastus lateralis muscle is located in the middle of the muscle belly, closer to its dorsal margin. Its area of pain projection reaches from the greater trochanter to the head of the fibula (▶ **Fig. 68.12**).

Trigger point 4: Trigger point 4 of the vastus lateralis muscle is located exactly in the middle of the muscle belly (▶ **Fig. 68.13**). It radiates along the femur up to the lateral gluteal region and the anterolateral knee joint region. The patella remains free of pain.

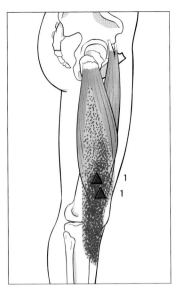

▶ **Fig. 68.10** Quadriceps femoris muscle (vastus lateralis muscle), trigger point 1.

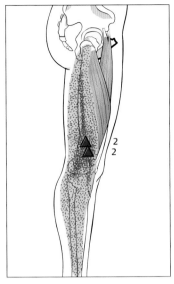

▶ **Fig. 68.11** Quadriceps femoris muscle (vastus lateralis muscle), trigger point 2.

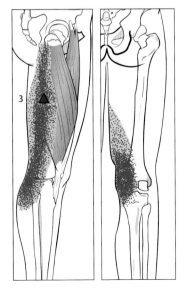

▶ **Fig. 68.12** Quadriceps femoris muscle (vastus lateralis muscle), trigger point 3.

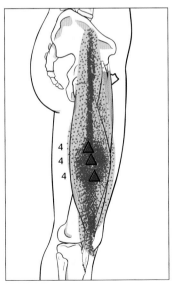

▶ **Fig. 68.13** Quadriceps femoris muscle (vastus lateralis muscle), trigger point 4.

Trigger point 5: Trigger point 5 of the vastus lateralis muscle is located directly below the greater trochanter, at the origin of the muscle. This is also its local area of pain radiation (▶ Fig. 68.14).

Knee Trigger Point

A nonmyogenic trigger point is located at the insertion of the lateral collateral ligament of the knee joint, with pain radiation into the lateral femoral condyle (▶ Fig. 68.15).

Important Acupuncture Points

▶ Fig. 68.16, ▶ Fig. 68.17

ST-31

Location: With the hip flexed, in a depression lateral to the sartorius muscle, at the intersection of a line connecting the anterior superior iliac spine with the lateral cranial pole of the patella and a horizontal line through the lower border of the symphysis.

ST-32

Location: 6 Cun above the upper lateral margin of the patella, on a line connecting the anterior superior iliac spine and the lateral cranial pole of the patella.

ST-33

Location: 3 Cun above the upper lateral margin of the patella, on a line connecting the anterior superior iliac spine and the lateral cranial pole of the patella.

ST-34

Location: With the knee slightly bent, 2 Cun above the upper lateral margin of the patella, in a depression of the vastus lateralis muscle. This point is located on a line connecting the anterior superior iliac spine and the lateral cranial pole of the patella.

ST-35

Location: With the knee slightly bent, below the patella and lateral to the patellar tendon.

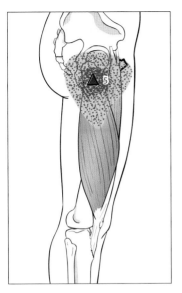

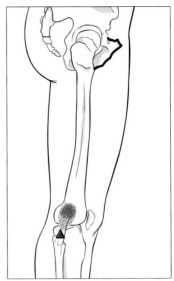

▶ **Fig. 68.14** Quadriceps femoris muscle (vastus lateralis muscle), trigger point 5.

▶ **Fig. 68.15** Quadriceps femoris muscle, knee trigger point.

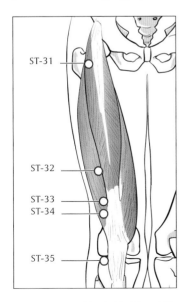

▶ **Fig. 68.16** ST-31, 32, 33, 34, and 35.

SP-10

Location: 2 Cun proximal to the medial cranial pole of the patella on the vastus medialis muscle, in a depression that is often easy to palpate. Another way to locate this point is to place the palm of the hand on the patella, with the thumb slightly abducted. SP-10 is located in front of the tip of the thumb.

SP-11

Location: 6 Cun above SP-10, lateral to the sartorius muscle, in a depression between this muscle and the vastus medialis muscle.

EX-LE-1 Kuangu (Hip Bone)

Location: Two points left and right, 1.5 Cun next to ST-34.

EX-LE-2 He Ding

Location: In the middle of the upper margin of the patella.

EX-LE-3 Baichonwo, Warm Nest

Location: 1 Cun above SP-10, in the region of the vastus medialis muscle.

EX-LE-4 Nei Xi Yan

Location: With the knee bent, in the depression medial to the patellar ligament, in the region of the inner "eye of the knee."

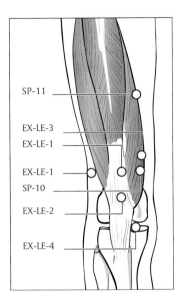

▶ **Fig. 68.17** SP-10, SP-11, EX-LE-1, EX-LE-2, EX-LE-3, and EX-LE-4.

69 Hamstring Muscles

Description of the Muscles

▶ Fig. 69.1, ▶ Fig. 69.2

Origin:
- Biceps muscle of the thigh, long head: tuberosity of ischium and sacrotuberal ligament
- Biceps muscle of the thigh, short head: linea aspera of the femur and lateral intermuscular septum
- Semimembranosus muscle: tuberosity of ischium, proximal and lateral to the common head
- Semitendinosus muscle: tuberosity of ischium

Insertion:
- Biceps muscle of the thigh: lateral surface of the head of the fibula and lateral condyle of the tibia
- Semimembranosus muscle: posteromedial part of the medial condyle of the tibia
- Semitendinosus muscle: medial surface of the tibia via the pes anserinus

Innervation:
- Biceps muscle of the thigh, long head: tibial division of sciatic nerve (L5–S2); short head: common peroneal division of sciatic nerve from nerve roots L5 to S2
- Semimembranosus and semitendinosus muscles: tibial division of sciatic nerve from nerve roots L5 to S2

Action: Powerful extension in the hip joint of the supporting leg; indirect flattening effect on lumbar lordosis. As an antagonist of the psoas muscle, it acts as a lateral rotator of the nonsupporting leg. The semimembranosus and semitendinosus muscles act as medial rotators.

Trigger Points of the Hamstring Muscles

Introduction: These trigger points are frequently found in athletes as a result of chronic strain, but also as a result of acute strain, for example, a 100-meter run.

Examination of trigger points: Targeted palpation of individual muscle portions, with the patient

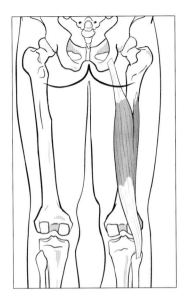

▶ **Fig. 69.1** Hamstring muscles (1).

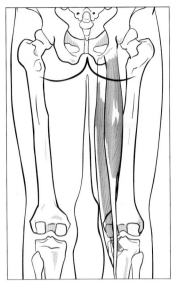

▶ **Fig. 69.2** Hamstring muscles (2).

preferably in a supine position and the hip joint mostly flexed. Treatment, on the other hand, is easiest with the patient in an abdominal position.

Trigger point therapy: These trigger points can be inactivated by dry-needling, without problems. Alternatively, conventional

needling or therapeutic local anesthesia are an option. Follow-up by the therapist involves stretching of the muscles with the patient in a supine position by flexing the hip joint with the leg extended. Patients can do this on their own in the supine position by actively extending the knee with the hip joint flexed.

Trigger Points and Pain Projection Areas

Biceps Muscle of the Thigh

These trigger points (▶ **Fig. 69.3**) are located at the transition from the middle to the distal third of the muscle. They cause radiation of pain into the popliteal fossa and into areas extending along the entire back of the thigh and down to the proximal region of the calf.

Semitendinosus and Semimembranosus Muscles

These trigger points (▶ **Fig. 69.4**) are located in the middle of the muscle belly, at the same level as those of the biceps muscle. They cause pain radiating to the origin (tuberosity of the ischium) and also along the entire postero-medial side of the thigh and the proximal portion of the lower leg.

Important Acupuncture Points

▶ Fig. 69.5

BL-36

Location: In the middle of the transverse gluteal fold.

BL-37

Location: On a line connecting BL-36 and BL-40, 6 Cun (two hand widths) distal to BL-36, or 1.5 Cun cranial to midway between BL-36 and BL-40.

BL-38

Location: 1 Cun cranial to BL-39 (1 Cun lateral to the middle of the popliteal fossa, medial to the tendon of the biceps muscle of the thigh).

BL-39

Location: 1 Cun lateral to the middle of the popliteal fossa, medial to the tendon of the biceps muscle of the thigh.

BL-40

Location: In the middle of the popliteal crease.

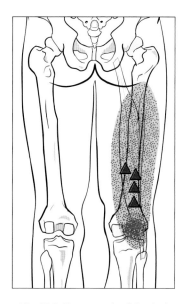

▶ **Fig. 69.3** Biceps muscle of the thigh, trigger points.

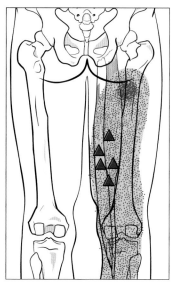

▶ **Fig. 69.4** Semitendinosus and semi-membranosus muscles, trigger points.

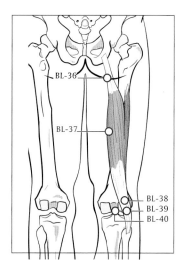

▶ **Fig. 69.5** BL-36, 37, 38, 39, and 40.

70 Gracilis Muscle

Description of the Muscle

▶ Fig. 70.1

Origin: Inferior ramus of pubic bone.

Insertion: Proximal end of the tibia, just below the medial epicondyle. (The tendons of the sartorius and semimembranosus muscles that insert anteriorly and posteriorly, respectively, combine with the tendon of the gracilis muscle to form the pes anserinus.)

Innervation: Anterior branch of the obturator nerve from nerve roots L2 to L4.

Action: Flexion of hip and knee joints; slight adduction of the thigh. With the knee joint flexed, medial rotation of the thigh.

Trigger Points

Introduction: Trigger points are frequently located in this area. It is somewhat difficult to differentiate this muscle from its surrounding structures. However, the trigger points are easy to locate.

Examination of trigger points: With the extended leg abducted, the muscle can be directly palpated in about the middle of its belly.

Trigger point therapy: These trigger points are easily inactivated by direct dry-needling. Follow-up treatment involves stretching the muscle by abducting the extended leg. This stretching technique is easy to learn and patients can perform it on their own.

Alternatively, conventional needling or therapeutic local anesthesia may be used.

As a further follow-up treatment, acu-taping (acupressure taping) is well suited to preventing relapses.

Trigger Points and Pain Projection Areas

The main trigger point (▶ Fig. 70.2) is located in the middle of the muscle belly. The pain radiates into the pubic symphysis and into the pes anserinus.

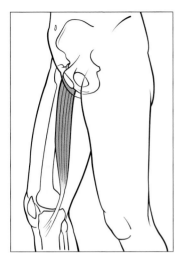

▶ **Fig. 70.1** Gracilis muscle.

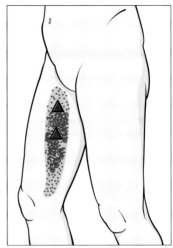

▶ **Fig. 70.2** Gracilis muscle, trigger points.

Important Acupuncture Points

▶ Fig. 70.3

LR-8

Location: LR-8 is located about 1 Cun cranial and ventral to KI-10, between the tendons of the semitendinosus and semimembranosus muscles and posterior to the medial epicondyle of the tibia. This point is located with the knee slightly flexed (and the knee supported by a cushion). It is located about 1 Cun proximal to the end of the popliteal crease.

LR-10

Location: About 3 Cun directly inferior to ST-30, at the lateral border of the abductor longus muscle (ST-30 is at the superior border of the pubic symphysis, 2 Cun lateral to the anterior median line).

SP-11

Location: 6 Cun superior to SP-10, lateral to the sartorius muscle, in a depression between this muscle and the vastus medialis muscle, on a line connecting SP-10 and SP-12.

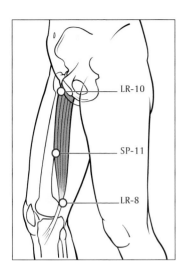

▶ **Fig. 70.3** LR-8, 10, and SP-11.

71 Tensor Muscle of the Fascia Lata

Description of the Muscle

▶ Fig. 71.1

Origin: Iliac crest, near the superior anterior iliac spine.

Insertion: Iliotibial tract in the middle third of the femur; the tract extends downward to the lateral condyle of the tibia.

Innervation: Superior gluteal nerve from the nerve root L4 to L5.

Action: Flexion and abduction of the thigh in the hip joint. This muscle is part of the accessory patellar ligament, which acts as reinforcement of the knee joint in case the quadriceps muscle of the thigh fails. Also a strong medial rotator of the hip joint.

Trigger Points

Introduction: Trigger points develop in this area in response to insufficiencies of the muscles linking the pelvis and trochanter.

They are also observed with chronic lumbosacral symptoms or with the onset of coxarthrosis.

These trigger points are often confused with trochanteric bursitis because the radiation of pain is similar.

Examination of trigger points: With the patient in a lateral position, provocation is successful when the muscle is palpated during extension, adduction, and lateral rotation.

Trigger point therapy: These trigger points can be deactivated without problems by dry-needling or therapeutic local anesthesia because there is no risk of damaging essential vessels or nerves. Follow-up treatment by stretching is done in the same position as for provocation. Additional trigger points might be present in the quadratus lumborum muscle or in the hip joint adductors, and their treatment should be considered.

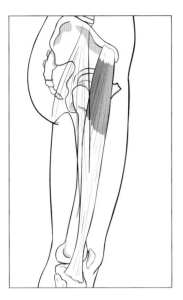

▶ **Fig. 71.1** Tensor Muscle of the fascia lata.

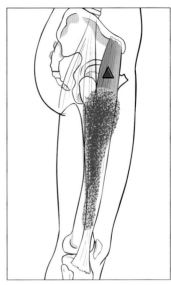

▶ **Fig. 71.2** Trigger points and pain projection areas.

Trigger Points and Pain Projection Areas

This trigger point (▶ **Fig. 71.2**) is located near the origin of the muscle in the proximal third of the muscle belly. The pain radiates caudally along the greater trochanter and to the middle third of the femur. Sometimes there are also trigger points along the fibula to the lateral ankle. In that case, radiation of pain may be confused with L5 symptoms.

Important Acupuncture Points

▶ Fig. 71.3

GB-29

Location: Midway between the anterior superior iliac spine and the most prominent site of the greater trochanter. This point is located with the hip joint flexed.

GB-31

Location: With the patient standing upright and the arm hanging down and fully extended, this point is located on the thigh at the tip of the middle finger, approximately in the region of the pant seam, 7 Cun cranial to the popliteal fold.

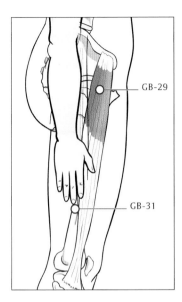

▶ **Fig. 71.3** GB-29 and 31.

72 Gastrocnemius Muscle

Description of the Muscle

▶ Fig. 72.1

Origin: Medial and lateral condyles of the femur.
Insertion: Cranial and medial portion of the tuberosity of calcaneus.
Innervation: Tibial nerve from the nerve roots S1 to S2.
Action: Strong flexion of the knee joint and the ankle joints. Also supinates the talocalcaneal joint.

Trigger Points

Introduction: These trigger points are frequently found in athletes, and also in cyclists due to fixation of the forefoot to the pedal. Patients report chronic symptoms of calf muscle strain. Latent trigger points may also cause spasms of the calf muscles at night.

Examination of trigger points: Local twitch responses can be induced in the trigger point regions in the proximal portion of the muscle bellies.

Trigger point therapy: These trigger points can be easily inactivated by dry-needling or conventional acupuncture, and also by therapeutic local anesthesia. Treatment is performed with the patient in the abdominal position.

Follow-up treatment by acu-taping is recommended.

Stretching can easily be carried out by the patients themselves. To achieve the best stretch effect on both heads of the gastrocnemius muscle, it is important to ensure that the foot is in sagittal alignment.

Trigger Points and Pain Projection Areas

▶ Fig. 72.2

Trigger point 1: Trigger point 1 is located in the medial head of the muscle in the proximal third of its belly. It leads to characteristic radiation of pain along the medial head of the muscle down to the palm of the foot. This may

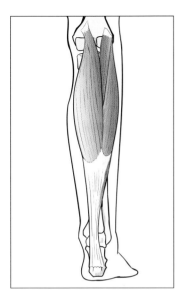

▶ **Fig. 72.1** Gastrocnemius muscle.

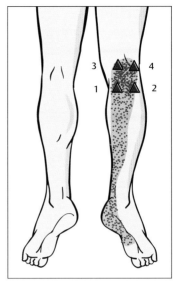

▶ **Fig. 72.2** Trigger points and pain projection areas.

cause it to be confused with calcaneal spur pain.

Trigger point 2: Trigger point 2 is located in the medial head of the muscle in the popliteal fossa and causes local radiation of pain.

Trigger point 3: Trigger point 3 is located in the lateral head of the muscle in the middle third of its belly and causes local radiation of pain.

Trigger Point 4: Trigger point 4 is located in the lateral head of the muscle, at the same level as trigger point 2, and causes local pain in the lateral portion of the popliteal fossa.

Important Acupuncture Points

▶ Fig. 72.3

BL-39

Location: 1 Cun lateral to the middle of the popliteal fossa, medial to the tendon of the biceps muscle of the thigh.

BL-40

Location: In the middle of the popliteal crease.

BL-57

Location: Halfway between BL-40 and BL-60; 8 Cun caudal to BL-40, in a depression between the bellies of the gastrocnemius muscle.

BL-58

Location: 1 Cun distal and lateral to BL-57, 7 Cun cranial to BL-60.

BL-60

Location: In the middle of a line connecting the highest protrusion of the lateral malleolus and the Achilles tendon (dorsal border).

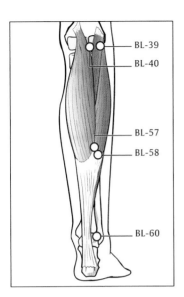

▶ **Fig. 72.3** BL-39, 40, 57, 58, and 60.

73 Anterior Tibial Muscle

▶ Fig. 73.1

Description of the Muscle

Origin: Lateral condyle of the tibia, proximal lateral half of the interosseous membrane of leg, deep crural fascia, and lateral intermuscular septum of leg.

Insertion: Medial and plantar surfaces of first cuneiform bone and also the base of first metatarsal bone.

Innervation: Deep peroneal nerve from the nerve root L4 to L5 (segment-indicating muscle of spinal cord segment L4).

Action: Extension of the ankle joints, raises the medial border of the foot (supination).

Trigger Points

Introduction: These trigger points are frequently activated by distortion of the muscle, but also by strain when running. In this context, fibular fracture or compartment syndrome should be considered for differential diagnosis.

Examination of trigger points: This muscle is easy to palpate. The trigger points are usually easily provoked by dorsiflexion and simultaneous pronation.

Trigger point therapy: Trigger point acupuncture should always be performed with the needle directed at an angle of 45° toward the lateral border of the tibia, to avoid damage to the anterior tibial artery and vein, and to the deep peroneal nerve.

Follow-up treatment involves stretching of the muscle in the direction of pain provocation.

Trigger Points and Pain Projection Areas

The main trigger point (▶ Fig. 73.2) is located in the proximal third of the muscle. It leads to characteristic radiation of pain along the muscle, with the greatest intensity over the ankle joints and the dorsal part of the big toe. Differential diagnosis may be complicated by possible confusion of these symptoms with irritation of the peroneal nerve or the spinal nerve root L5.

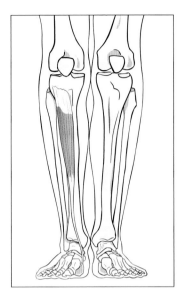

▶ **Fig. 73.1** Anterior tibial muscle.

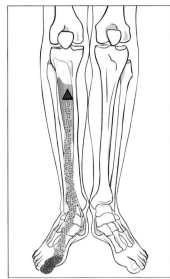

▶ **Fig. 73.2** Anterior tibial muscle, trigger point.

Important Acupuncture Points

▶ Fig. 73.3

ST-35

Location: With knee slightly flexed, inferior to the patella and lateral to the patellar tendon; the lateral "eye of the knee" (i.e., the points below it, medial and lateral to the patella).

The lateral "eye of the knee" corresponds to point ST-35, the medial "eye of the knee" corresponds to the extra point Xi Yan EX-LE-5.

ST-36

Location: With knee slightly flexed, 3 Cun inferior to ST-35, at about the level of the inferior boundary of the tuberosity of the tibia, about one width of the middle finger lateral to the anterior border of the tibia, in the tibialis anterior muscle.

ST-37

Location: 3 Cun distal to ST-36 and one width of the middle finger lateral to the anterior border of the tibia, in the tibialis anterior muscle.

ST-38

Location: At the midpoint of a line connecting ST-35 and ST-41, about one width of the middle finger lateral to the anterior border of the tibia or 2 Cun caudal to ST-37.

ST-39

Location: 1 Cun inferior to ST-38 and one width of the middle finger lateral to the anterior border of the tibia.

ST-40

Location: One width of the middle finger lateral to ST-38.

ST-41

Location: In the anterior middle of the line connecting the lateral malleolus with the medial malleolus, between the tendons of the long extensor muscle of the big toe and the long extensor muscle of the toes, over the upper ankle joint.

EX-LE-7

Location: On the Stomach Channel, 2 Cun distal to ST-36.

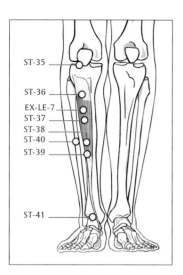

▶ **Fig. 73.3** ST-35, 36, 37, 38, 39, 40, 41, and EX-LE-7.

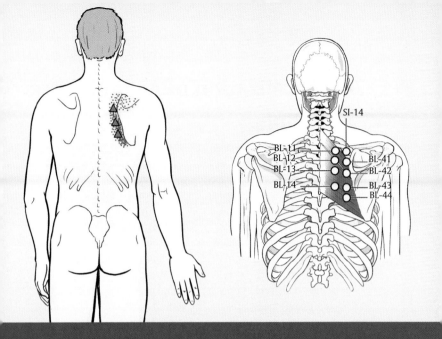

Part 4
Appendix

74 Localization of Acupuncture Points

In China, acupuncture points are primarily localized using proportional measurements expressed in **body Cun**. The unit of measurement, Cun, is further divided into Fen, such that 1 Cun equals 10 Fen.

For various body regions, proportional measurements are given in Cun. For example, the distance between the elbow crease and wrist measures 12 Cun. In the lower arm region, specifications in Cun are always made according to these proportional measurements given as a total number of Cun. For example, a distance of 4 Cun from the dorsal wrist crease means that the point lies proximal to the wrist crease at one-third of the total distance between the elbow crease and wrist.

This proportional orientation takes into account individual variations in body proportions. This is of particular importance in the abdominal region. For example, 1 Cun cranial to the symphysis does not mean that the point (CV-3) is found one width of a patient's thumb above the symphysis. Instead, the total distance between the navel and upper margin of the symphysis has to be subdivided into five equal sections (e.g., by using a graded rubber band as a measuring tape). The point to be localized lies proximal to one-fifth of the total distance between the navel and upper margin of the symphysis. Only if orientation according to proportional measurements in **body Cun** is not feasible, is the patient's **thumb Cun** used as a unit of measurement.

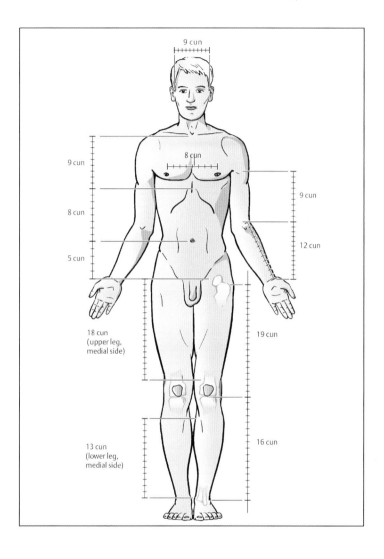

Proportional Measurement Based on Body Cun

Face

The distance between both Points ST-8 measures 9 Cun.

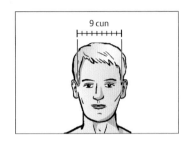

Thorax

The distance between the manubrium of the sternum and base of the xiphoid process measures 9 Cun. However, orientation in the thoracic region is based on intercostal space (ICS). The transition between sternal manubrium and sternal body is clearly palpable in the area of the sternal synchondrosis. The second rib lies lateral to this transition. The second ICS lies caudal to the second rib.

The distance between the two mamilla measures 8 Cun.

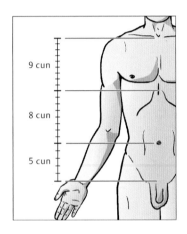

Abdomen

The distance between the base of the xiphoid process and the navel measures 8 Cun.

The distance between the navel and upper margin of the symphysis measures 5 Cun.

Upper Extremity

The distance between the elbow crease and the upper fold of the armpit measures 9 Cun.

The distance between the elbow crease and palmar wrist crease measures 12 Cun.

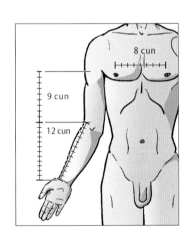

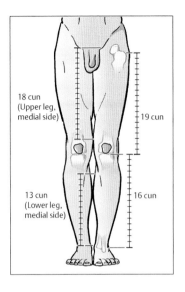

18 cun
(Upper leg,
medial side)

19 cun

13 cun
(Lower leg,
medial side)

16 cun

Lower Extremity

Lateral side: The distance between the highest point of the greater trochanter and the knee-joint crevice (lower edge of patella) measures 19 Cun.

The distance between the knee-joint crevice and the highest point of the lateral malleolus measures 16 Cun.

Medial side: The distance between the upper margin of the symphysis and the transition of the femoral shaft to the medial epicondyle measures 18 Cun.

The distance between the transition of the tibial shaft to the medial condyle of the tibia and the medial malleolus measures 13 Cun.

Dorsal Body

The distance between both mastoid processes measures 9 Cun.

The distance between the dorsal midline through the spinous processes and medial margin of the scapula at the attachment of the scapular spine measures 3 Cun (in a patient with arms hanging down).

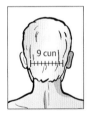

9 cun

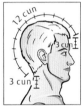

12 cun

3 cun

3 cun

Lateral Head

The distance between the middle of the frontal hairline and the middle of the dorsal hairline measures 12 Cun.

The distance between the middle of the eyebrow and the frontal hairline measures 3 Cun.

The distance between the spinous process of C7 and the dorsal hairline measures 3 Cun.

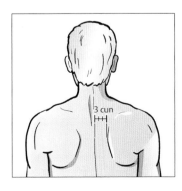

3 cun

Proportional Measurement Based on Finger Cun

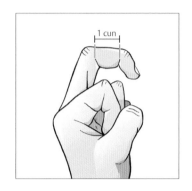

The distance between the palmar crease of the proximal interphalangeal joint and the palmar crease of the distal interphalangeal joint of the middle finger measures 1 Cun.

At its greatest width, the thumb measures 1 Cun.

Middle and index fingers together measure 1.5 Cun in the most distal region.

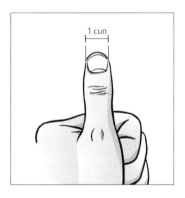

Middle, index, and ring fingers together measure 2 Cun in the most distal region. Middle, index, ring, and little fingers together measure 3 Cun in the widest area over the knuckles.

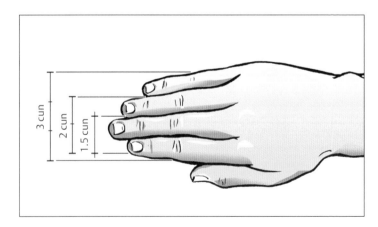

75 References

[1] Academy of Traditional Chinese Medicine. Essentials of Chinese Acupuncture. Beijing: Foreign Languages; 1980

[2] Academy of Traditional Chinese Medicine. An Outline of Chinese Acupuncture. Beijing: Foreign Languages; 1975

[3] Amano M, Umeda G, Nakajima H, Yatsuki K. Characteristics of work actions of shoe manufacturing assembly line workers and a cross-sectional factor-control study on occupational cervicobrachial disorders. Sangyo Igaku. 1988; 30 (1):3–12

[4] Andersen JH, Kaergaard A, Rasmussen K. Myofascial pain in different occupational groups with monotonous repetitive work (abstract). J Musculoskeletal Pain. 1995; 3(suppl 1):57

[5] Bachmann G. Die Akupunktur—eine Ordnungstherapie. Vol 1. 3rd ed. Heidelberg: Haug; 1980

[6] Bahr FR. Einführung in die wissenschaftliche Akupunktur. 6th ed. Braunschweig: Vieweg; 1995

[7] Bahr RR, Reis A, Straube EM, et al. Skriptum für die Aufbaustufe aller Akupunkturverfahren. 4th ed. Deutsche Akademie für Akupunktur + Auriculomedizin e.V. München: Eigenverlag; 1993

[8] Baker BA. The muscle trigger: evidence of overload injury. J Neurol Orthop Med Surg. 1986; 7(1):35–44

[9] Basmajian JV. New views on muscular tone and relaxation. Can Med Assoc J. 1957; 77(3):203–205

[10] Bergsmann O, Bergsmann R. Projektionssyndrome. Vienna: Facultas; 1988

[11] Bergsmann O, Bergsmann R. Projektionssymptome. 4th ed. Vienna: Facultas; 1997

[12] Bischko J. Einführung in die Akupunktur. Vol. 1. 3rd ed. Heidelberg: Haug; 1989

[13] Bischko J. Akupunktur für mäßig Fortgeschrittene. Vol. 2. Heidelberg: Haug; 1985

[14] Bischko J, ed. Weltkongress für wissenschaftliche Akupunktur. Kongreßband. Part 1. Vienna: 1983

[15] Bischko J. Sonderformen der Akupunktur. Broschüre 21.4.0. aus dem Handbuch der Akupunktur und Aurikulotherapie. Heidelberg: Haug; 1981

[16] Bogduk N, Jull G. Die Pathophysiolgie der akuten LWS-Blockierung. Manuelle Medizin. 1985; 23:77–81

[17] Bolten W, Kempel-Waibel A, Pför-
ringer W. Analyse der Krankheit-
skosten bei Rückenschmerzen.
Medizinische Klinik. 1998; 93
(6):388–393

[18] Bossy J, Maurel JC, Godlewski G.
[Macroscopic substratum of acu-
puncture points]. Bull Assoc Anat
(Nancy). 1975; 59(165):357–362

[19] Bucek R. Lehrbuch der Ohrakupunktur. Eine Synopsis der franzö-
sischen, chinesischen und
russischen Schulen. Heidelberg:
Haug; 1994

[20] Chen J, ed. Anatomical Atlas of
Chinese Acupuncture Points.
Jinan: Shandong Science and
Technology; 1982

[21] Chen Q, Bensamoun S, Basford JR,
Thompson JM, An KN. Identification and quantification of myofascial taut bands with magnetic
resonance elastography. Arch Phys
Med Rehabil. 2007; 88(12):1658–
1661

[22] Chinese Traditional Medical Col-
lege and Chinese Traditional Medical Research Institute of Shanghai.
Anatomical Charts of the Acupuncture Points and 14 Meridians.
Shanghai: People's Publishing
House; 1976

[23] Cho ZH, Hwang SC, Wong EK,
et al. Neural substrates, experi-
mental evidences and functional
hypothesis of acupuncture mechanisms. Acta Neurol Scand. 2006;
113(6):370–377

[24] DÄGfA. Akupunktur. Skripten
Grundkurs I–III. 1995

[25] Dejung B. [The treatment of
"chronic strains."]. Schweiz Z
Sportmed. 1988; 36(4):161–168

[26] Dejung B, Gröbli C, Colla F, et al.
Triggerpunkt-Therapie. 2nd ed.
Bern: Hans Huber; 2006

[27] Dommerholt J, Norris RN. Physical
Therapy Management of the
Instrumental Musician. In: Gal-
lagher SP, ed. Physical Therapy for
Performing Artists. Part II: Music
and Dance. Philadelphia: Saun-
ders; 1997

[28] Dung HC. Anatomical features
contributing to the formation of
acupuncture points. Am J Acupunct. 1984; 12(2):139–143

[29] Egle ET, Hoffmann SO, Nickel R.
Psychoanalytisch orientierte Ther-
apieverfahren bei Schmerz. In:
Basler HD, et al, eds. Psychologi-
sche Schmerztherapie. 5th ed.
Heidelberg: Springer; 2003

[30] Elias J. Lehr- und Praxisbuch der
Ohrakupunktur. Tenningen:
Sommer; 1990

[31] Ettlin TM, Kaeser HM. Muskelver-
spannungen: Ätiologie, Diagnostik
und Therapie. Stuttgart: Thieme;
1998

[32] Flows B. Der wirkungsvolle Aku-
punkturpunkt. Kötzting: VGM;
1993

[33] Frick H, Leonhardt H, Starck D. All-
gemeine Anatomie. Spezielle
Anatomie I, II. Taschenbuch der
gesamten Anatomie. Vols. 1, 2.
3rd ed. Stuttgart: Thieme; 1987

[34] Gerhard I. Die Ohrakupunktur. Technik und Einsatz in der Gynäkologie sowie Ergebnis bei Sterilitätsbehandlung. Erfahrungsheilkunde. 1990; 39:503–511

[35] Gerhard I, Müller C. Akupunktur in der Gynäkologie und Geburtshilfe. In: Dittmer FW, Loch EG, Wiesenauer M, eds. Naturheilverfahren in der Frauenheilkunde und Geburtshilfe. 3rd ed. Stuttgart: Hippokrates; 2003

[36] Gerhard I, Poostnek F. Möglichkeiten der Therapie durch Ohrakupunktur bei weiblicher Sterilität. Geburtshilfe Frauenheilkd. 1988; 48:154–171

[37] Gleditsch JM. Reflexzonen und Somatotopien als Schlüssel zu einer Gesamtschau des Menschen. 3rd ed. Schorndorf: WBV Biologisch-Medizinische Verlagsgesellschaft; 1988

[38] Gongwang L, ed. Acupoints and Meridians. Beijing: Huaxia Publishing House; 1996

[39] Gray H, et al. Gray's Anatomy. 41st ed. Amsterdam: Elsevier; 2015

[40] Grosjean B, Dejung B. [Achillodynia—an unsolvable problem?]. Schweiz Z Sportmed. 1990; 38 (1):17–24

[41] Gunn CC. The Gunn Approach to the Treatment of Chronic Pain. New York: Churchill Livingstone; 1996

[42] Hasenbring M. Biopsychosoziale Grundlagen der Chronifizierung. In: Zenz M, Jurna I, eds. Lehrbuch der Schmerztherapie. 2nd ed. Stuttgart: Wissenschaftliche Verlagsgesellschaft; 2001

[43] Hecker HU. VISDAK, Visuell-didaktisches System – eine kombinierte Darstellung von Bild und Text auf dem Gebiet der Akupunktur und Naturheilkunde. Anmeldung Deutsches Patentamt München; 1997

[44] Hecker HU, Liebchen K, eds. Aku-Taping. Akupunkturpunkte, viszerale und myofasziale Triggerpunkte. Stuttgart: Haug; 2012

[45] Hecker HU, Steveling A, Peuker ET. Microsystems Acupuncture. The Complete Guide: Ear–Scalp–Mouth–Hand. Stuttgart: Thieme; 2005

[46] Hecker HU, Steveling A, Peuker ET, Kaster J. Practice of Acupuncture. Point Location–Treatment Options–TCM Basics. Stuttgart: Thieme; 2004

[47] Heine H. Anatomische Struktur der Akupunkturpunkte. Dtsch Z Akup. 1988; 31:26–30

[48] Helms JM. Acupuncture for the management of primary dysmenorrhea. Obstet Gynecol. 1987; 69 (1):51–56

[49] Hides JA, Jull GA, Richardson CA. Long-term effects of specific stabilizing exercises for first-episode low back pain. Spine. 2001; 26 (11):E243–E248

[50] Hinkelthein E, Zalpour C. Diagnose- und Therapiekonzepte in

der Osteopathie. Heidelberg: Springer; 2005

[51] Hirayama J, Takahashi Y, Nakajima Y, Takahashi K, Yamagata M, Moriya H. Effects of electrical stimulation of the sciatic nerve on background electromyography and static stretch reflex activity of the trunk muscles in rats: possible implications of neuronal mechanisms in the development of sciatic scoliosis. Spine. 2001; 26 (6):602–609

[52] Hubbard DR, Berkoff GM. Myofascial trigger points show spontaneous needle EMG activity. Spine. 1993; 18(13):1803–1807

[53] Hünting W, Läubli T, Grandjean E. Postural and visual loads at VDT workplaces. I. Constrained postures. Ergonomics. 1981; 24 (12):917–931

[54] International Anatomical Nomenclature Committee. Nomina anatomica. 6th ed. Edinburgh: Churchill Livingstone; 1989

[55] Janda V. Manuelle Muskelfunktionsdiagnostik. 3rd ed. Munich: Elsevier; 2000

[56] Jull G, Barrett C, Magee R, Ho P. Further clinical clarification of the muscle dysfunction in cervical headache. Cephalalgia. 1999; 19 (3):179–185

[57] Junghanns KH. Akupunktur in der Geburtshilfe und Frauenheilkunde —ein Naturheilverfahren als "sanfte Alternative." Erfahrungsheilkunde. 1993; 3:114–123

[58] Junghanns KH. Akupunktur in der Geburtshilfe und Gynäkologie Bereicherung der Therapiemöglichkeiten. Therapiewoche. 1992; 43(50):2715–2720

[59] Junghanns KH. Akupunktur in der Geburtshilfe—Behandlungsmöglichkeiten am Beispiel der Ohrakupunktur. Gyn.-Praktische Gynäkologie 1997;434–450

[60] Kampik G. Propädeutik der Akupunktur. 4th ed. Stuttgart: Hippokrates; 2000

[61] Kantoner militärsan. Einheit. Zhen Jiu Xue Wei Gua Tu Shuo Mind. Volksgesundheitsverlag der VR China

[62] Kapandji IA. Funktionelle Anatomie der Gelenke. 4th ed. Stuttgart: Thieme; 2006

[63] Kawakita K, Shinbara H, Imai K, Fukuda F, Yano T, Kuriyama K. How do acupuncture and moxibustion act? Focusing on the progress in Japanese acupuncture research. J Pharmacol Sci. 2006; 100(5):443–459

[64] Kendall F, Kendall E. Muskeln, Funktion und Test. 2nd ed. Stuttgart: G. Fischer; 1988

[65] Kendall F, Kendall E. Muscles, Testing and Function. 3rd ed. Baltimore: Williams & Wilkins; 1983

[66] Kikaldy-Willis WH. Managing Low Back Pain. New York: Churchill Livingstone; 1988

[67] Kitzinger E. Der Akupunktur-Punkt. 2nd ed. Vienna: Maudrich; 1995

[68] König G, Wancura L. Neue chinesi-sche Akupunktur. 6th ed. Vienna: Maudrich; 1996

[69] König G, Wancura L. Einführung in die chinesische Ohrakupunktur. 9th ed. Heidelberg: Haug; 1989

[70] König G, Wancura L. Praxis und Theorie der Neuen chinesischen Akupunktur. Vol. 1, 2. Vienna: Maudrich; 1979/1983

[71] Kropej H. Systematik der Ohraku-punktur. 7th ed. Heidelberg: Haug; 1997

[72] Kuan TS, Hong CZ, Chen JT, Chen SM, Chien CH. The spinal cord connections of the myofascial trig-ger spots. Eur J Pain. 2007; 11 (6):624–634

[73] Kubiena G, Meng A. Die neuen Extrapunkte in der chinesischen Akupunktur. Vienna: Maudrich; 1994

[74] Kubiena G, Meng A, Petricek E, et al. Handbuch der Akupunktur—der traditionell chinesische und der moderne Weg. Vienna: Orac; 1991

[75] Lang J. Klinische Anatomie des Kopfes. Berlin: Springer; 1981

[76] Lange G. Akupunktur in der Ohr-muschel. Diagnostik und Therapie. Schorndorf: WBV Biologisch-Medi-zinische Verlagsgesellschaft; 1985

[77] Langevin HM, Churchill DL, Wu J, et al. Evidence of connective tissue involvement in acupuncture. FASEB J. 2002; 16(8):872–874

[78] Lanz TV, Wachsmuth W. Prakti-sche Anatomie. Ein Lehr- und Hilfsbuch der anatomischen Grundlagen ärztlichen Handelns. Berlin: Springer; 1993–1996

[79] Lin TY, Teixeira MJ, et al. Work-related Musculo-skeletal Disor-ders. In: Fischer AA, ed. Myo-fas-cial Pain, Update in Diagnosis and Treatment. Philadelphia: Saun-ders; 1997

[80] Maciocia G. The Foundations of Chinese Medicine. New York: Churchill Livingstone; 1989

[81] Marx HG. Medikamentfreie Entgif-tung von Suchtkranken—Bericht über den Einsatz der Akupunktur. Suchtgefahren. 1984; 30

[82] Maurer-Groeli YA. Weichteilrheu-matismus bei Depression. Akt Rheumatol. 1978; 3:123–128

[83] McNulty WH, Gevirtz RN, Hub-bard DR, Berkoff GM. Needle elec-tromyographic evaluation of trigger point response to a psy-chological stressor. Psychophysiol-ogy. 1994; 31(3):313–316

[84] Mense S. Pathophysiologie der Muskelverspannungen. In: Ettlin TM, Kaeser HE, eds. Muskelver-spannungen. Stuttgart: Thieme; 1998

[85] Mense S, Simons DG, Russell IJ. Muscle Pain. Understanding its Nature, Diagnosis and Treatment. Philadelphia: Lippincott Williams & Wilkins; 2001

[86] Middlekauff HR. Acupuncture in the treatment of heart failure. Cardiol Rev. 2004; 12(3):171–173

[87] Müller-Ehrenberg H, Licht G. Diagnostik und Therapie von myofaszialen Schmerzsyndromen mittels der fokussierten stosswelle ESWT. MOT. 2005; 5:75–78

[88] Nogier PM. Lehrbuch der Aurikulotherapie. Saint-Ruffine: Maisonneuve; 1969

[89] Nogier R. Auriculotherapy. Stuttgart: Thieme: 2008

[90] Ogata A, Sugenoya J, Nishimura N, Matsumoto T. Low and high frequency acupuncture stimulation inhibits mental stress-induced sweating in humans via different mechanisms. Auton Neurosci. 2005; 118(1–2):93–101

[91] O'Sullivan PB, Phyty GD, Twomey LT, Allison GT. Evaluation of specific stabilizing exercise in the treatment of chronic low back pain with radiologic diagnosis of spondylolysis or spondylolisthesis. Spine. 1997; 22(24):2959–2967

[92] Paoletti S. Faszien. Munich: Urban & Fischer; 2001

[93] Petricek E, Zeitler H. Neue systematische Ordnung der NeuPunkte. Heidelberg: Haug; 1976

[94] Peuker E, Cummings M. Anatomy for the acupuncturist—facts and fiction; 1: The head and neck region. Acupunct Med 2003; 21: 2–8; 2: The chest, abdomen, and back. Acupunct Med 2003; 21: 72–9; 3: Upper and lower extremity. Acupunct Med. 2003; 21:122–132

[95] Peuker ET, Filler TJ. The innervation of the external ear. Clin Anat. 2001:14

[96] Peuker ET, Filler TJ. Forensische Aspekte der Akupunktur – Eine Übersicht vor dem Hintergrund anatomischer Grundlagen. Ärztezeitschrift für Naturheilverfahren. 1997; 38:833–842

[97] Peuker ET, Filler TJ. The need for practical courses in anatomy for acupuncturists. FACT. 1997; 2(4):194

[98] Plummer JP. Anatomical findings at acupuncture loci. Am J Chin Med. 1980; 8(1–2):170–180

[99] Pongratz DE, Späth M. Morphologic aspects of muscle pain syndromes—a critical review. Phys Med Rehabil Clin N Am. 1997; 8 (1):55–68

[100] Pöntinen PJ, Gleditsch J, Pothmann R. Triggerpunkte und Triggermechanismen. 3rd ed. Stuttgart: Hippokrates; 2005

[101] Pothmann R, ed. Akupunktur-Repetitorium. 3rd ed. Stuttgart: Hippokrates; 1997

[102] Rampes H, Peuker ET. Adverse effects of acupuncture. In: Ernst E, White A, eds. Acupuncture: a Scientific Appraisal. Woburn, MA: Butterworth-Heinemann; 1999

[103] Raspe H, Kohlmann T. Die aktuelle Rückenschmerzentherapie. In: Pfingsten M, Hildebrandt J, eds. Chronischer Rückenschmerz. Bern: Huber; 1998

[104] Raspe H, Kohlmann T. Kreuzsch-
merzen (3): Rückenschmerzen—
eine Epidemie unserer Tage?
Dtsch Arztebl. 1993; 90
(44):2165–2172

[105] Rauber A, Kopsch F. In: von H.
Leonhardt, B. Tillmann, G. Töndury, et al, eds. Anatomie des
Menschen. Lehrbuch und Atlas.
20th ed. Stuttgart: Thieme; 1987

[106] Richardson C, Jull G, et al. Therapeutic Exercise for Spinal Segmental Stabilization in Low Back Pain:
Scientific Basis and Clinical
Approach. London: Churchill Livingstone; 1999

[107] Richter K, Becke H. Akupunktur.
Tradition, Theorie, Praxis. 2nd ed.
Berlin: Ullstein-Mosby; 1995

[108] Richter P, Hebgen E. Trigger Points
and Muscle Chains in Osteopathy.
Stuttgart: Thieme; 2008

[109] Rohen J. Topographische Anatomie. 10th ed. Stuttgart: Schattauer; 2000

[110] Rohen J. Funktionelle Anatomie
des Menschen. 5th ed. Stuttgart:
Schattauer; 1987

[111] Rohen J. Funktionelle Anatomie
des Nervensystems. 4th ed. Stuttgart: Schattauer; 1985

[112] Rosen NB. Myofascial pain: the
great mimicker and potentiator of
other diseases in the performing
artist. Md Med J. 1993; 42
(3):261–266

[113] Rubach A. Principles of Ear Acupuncture. Stuttgart: Thieme; 2016

[114] Schmidt H. Konstitutionelle Akupunkturpunkte. Stuttgart: Hippokrates; 1988

[115] Schnorrenberger CC. Die topogra-
phisch-anatomischen Grundlagen
der chinesischen Akupunktur und
Ohrakupunktur. 6th ed. Stuttgart:
Hippokrates; 1994

[116] Schnorrenberger CC. Lehrbuch
der chinesischen Medizin für west-
liche Ärzte. Die theoretischen
Grundlagen der chinesischen Akupunktur und Arzneiverordnung.
3rd ed. Stuttgart: Hippokrates;
1985

[117] Schwind P. Faszien- und Membran-
technik. Munich: Urban & Fischer;
2003

[118] Shah JP, Danoff JV, Desai MJ, et al.
Biochemicals associated with pain
and inflammation are elevated in
sites near to and remote from
active myofascial trigger points.
Arch Phys Med Rehabil. 2008; 89
(1):16–23

[119] Shah JP, Phillips TM, Danoff JV,
Gerber LH. An in vivo microanalyt-
ical technique for measuring the
local biochemical milieu of human
skeletal muscle. J Appl Physiol
(1985). 2005; 99(5):1977–1984

[120] Sikdar S, Shah JP, Gilliams E,
Gebreab T, Gerber LH. Assess-
ment of myofascial trigger points
(MTrPs): a new application of
ultrasound imaging and vibration
sonoelastography. Conf Proc IEEE
Eng Med Biol Soc. 2008;
2008:5585–5588

[121] Silverstein BA. The prevalence of upper extremity cumulative trauma disorders in industry. Ann Arbor: University of Michigan; 1985

[122] Simons DG, Travell JG, Simons LS. Myofascial pain and dysfunction. Baltimore: Williams & Wilkins; 1999

[123] Sobotta J, Becher H. Atlas der Anatomie des Menschen. Vol. 2. In: Ferner von H, Staubesand J, eds. Brust, Bauch, Becken, untere Extremität. 19th ed. Munich: Urban & Schwarzenberg; 1988

[124] State Standard of the People's Republic of China. The Location of Acupoints. Beijing (VR China): Foreign Languages; 1990

[125] Strauß K, ed. Akupunktur in der Suchtmedizin. 2nd ed. Stuttgart: Hippokrates; 1999

[126] Strittmatter B. Ear Acupuncture. A Precise Pocket Atlas Based on the Works of Nogier/Bahr. 2nd ed. Stuttgart: Thieme; 2011

[127] Stux G, Stiller N, Pomeranz B. Akupunktur—Lehrbuch und Atlas. 6th ed. Berlin: Springer; 2003

[128] Taylor LS, Porter BC, Rubens DJ, Parker KJ. Three-dimensional sonoelastography: principles and practices. Phys Med Biol. 2000; 45 (6):1477–1494

[129] Thali A, et al. Die Rolle psychosozialer Faktoren bei protrahierten und invalidisierenden Verläufen nach Traumatisierungen im unteren Wirbelsäulenbereich. Bellikon: Suva-Klinik; 1993

[130] Tillmann B. Farbatlas der Anatomie. Stuttgart: Thieme; 1997

[131] Tittel K. Beschreibende und funktionelle Anatomie des Menschen. 14th ed. Stuttgart: G. Fischer; 2003

[132] Töndury G. Angewandte und topographische Anatomie. 5th ed. Stuttgart: Thieme; 1981

[133] Travell JG, Simons DG. Myofascial Pain and Dysfunction. Vol. 1, 2. Baltimore: Williams & Wilkins; 1992

[134] Turo D, Otto P, Shah JP, et al. Ultrasonic tissue characterization of the upper trapezius muscle in patients with myofascial pain syndrome. Conf Proc IEEE Eng Med Biol Soc. 2012; 2012:4386–4389

[135] Überall MA, et al. DGS-Praxisleitlinie Tumorbedingte Durchbruchschmerzen. www.dgs-praxisleitlinien.de

[136] Umlauf R. Zu den wissenschaftlichen Grundlagen der Aurikulotherapie. Dtsch Z Akup. 1989; 3:59–65

[137] Van Nghi N. Pathogenese und Pathologie der Energetik in der chinesischen Medizin. Vol. 1, 2. Uelzen: Medizinisch-Literarische Verlagsgesellschaft mbH; 1989/90

[138] Walsh EG. Muscles, Masses and Motion—The Physiology of Normality, Hypotonicity, Spasticity and Rigidity. Oxford: McKeith Press, Blackwell; 1992

[139] Webster BS, Snook SH. The cost of 1989 workers' compensation low back pain claims. Spine. 1994; 19 (10):1111–1115, discussion 1116

[140] Xinnong C. Chinese Acupuncture and Moxibustion. 3rd ed. Foreign Languages Press; 2009

[141] Yelin EH, Felts WR. A summary of the impact of musculoskeletal conditions in the United States. Arthritis Rheum. 1990; 33 (5):750–755

76 Illustration Credits

Figs. 2.1, 2.2, 3.1, 3.2, 4.1, 4.2, 5.1, 5.2, 6.1, 6.2, 7.1, 7.2, 7.3, 8.1, 8.2, 8.3, 9.1, 9.2, 9.3, 10.1, 10.2, 11.1, 11.2, 12.1, 12.2, 12,3, 13.1, 13.2, 14.1, 15.1, 15.2 from Steveling A, Hecker HU, Peuker ET. Repetitorium Akupunktur. Stuttgart: Hippokrates; 2010.

Fig. 39.1 from Richter P, Hebgen E. Triggerpunkte und Muskelfunktionsketten. 3rd ed. Stuttgart: Haug; 2011, p. 136.

Fig. 39.2 from Agarwal K, ed. Ganzheitliche Schmerztherapie. Stuttgart: Haug; 2013, p. 104 (© Dr. med. Elmar T. Peuker, Münster, Germany).

Fig. 39.3 from Dejung B. Triggerpunkt-Therapie. 3rd ed. Bern: Huber; 2009.

Figs. 39.4 and 39.5 from Gautschi R. Manuelle Triggerpunkt-Therapie. 2nd ed. Stuttgart: Thieme; 2013.

Fig. 39.6 from Hecker HU, Liebchen K, eds. Aku-Taping. Stuttgart: Haug; 2012, p. 30, Fig. 2.5.

All other illustrations from Hecker HU, Steveling A, Peuker ET, Kastner J, Liebchen K. Taschenlehrbuch der Akupunktur. 3rd ed. Stuttgart: Hippokrates; 2007.

Body Points

Ear Points

Trigger Points

General Index